*David J. Bellis*

# Hotel Ritz—
# Comparing Mexican
# and U.S. Street Prostitutes
## *Factors in HIV/AIDS*
## *Transmission*

# Hotel Ritz—
# Comparing Mexican
# and U.S. Street Prostitutes
## *Factors in HIV/AIDS*
## *Transmission*

## Haworth Psychosocial Issues of HIV/AIDS
### R. Dennis Shelby, PhD
### Senior Editor

# Hotel Ritz—
# Comparing Mexican
# and U.S. Street Prostitutes
## *Factors in HIV/AIDS Transmission*

David J. Bellis

The Haworth Press®
New York • London • Oxford

The Haworth Press, Inc., 10 Alice Street, Binghamton, NY 13904-1580.

PUBLISHER'S NOTE
Names of study participants discussed or quoted in this book have been changed to protect confidentiality.

Cover design by Lora Wiggins.

**Library of Congress Cataloging-in-Publication Data**

Bellis, David J., 1944-
    Hotel ritz—comparing Mexican and U.S. street prostitutes : factors in HIV/AIDS transmission / David J. Bellis.
        p. cm.
Includes bibliographical references and index.
    ISBN 0-7890-1775-X (hard cover : alk. paper) — ISBN 0-7890-1776-8 (soft cover : alk. paper)
    1. AIDS (Disease)—California, Southern. 2. Prostitutes—Diseases—California, Southern. 3. Prostitutes—Drug use—California, Southern. 4. Heroin habit—California, Southern. 5. AIDS (Disease)—Mexico. 6. Prostitutes—Diseases—Mexico. 7. Prostitutes—Drug use—Mexico. 8. Heroin habit—Mexico.
    [DNLM: 1. HIV Infections—transmission—Mexico. 2. HIV Infections—transmission—United States. 3. Acquired Immunodeficiency Syndrome—transmission—Mexico. 4. Acquired Immunodeficiency Syndrome—transmission—United States. 5. Prostitution—Mexico. 6. Prostitution—United States. 7. Sex Behavior—Mexico. 8. Sex Behavior—United States. 9. Sexually Transmitted Diseases—prevention & control—Mexico. 10. Sexually Transmitted Diseases—prevention & control—United States. 11. Substance-Related Disorders—epidemiology—Mexico. 12. Substance-Related Disorders—epidemiology—United States. WC 503.3 B444h 2002]. I. Title.

RA643.84.C2 B455 2002
362.1'969792—dc21
                                                                                                    2002015321

To my parents, my wife Ann, my son James,
and my mentor, Bill Wilson

# ABOUT THE AUTHOR

**David J. Bellis, PhD,** has taught at USC, UCLA, Long Beach State University, and Long Beach City College. He has been a professor at California State University in San Bernardino since 1985, where he chairs the public administration department. He is the recipient of the American Society for Public Administration's Outstanding Educator Award and 11 awards from California State University for outstanding research and teaching. His professional work spans 32 years of developing, managing, and evaluating over 35 narcotic addiction treatment, gang violence reduction, and delinquency prevention programs.

Dr. Bellis has treated over 10,000 heroin addicts and consulted to California agencies including the State Department of Corrections, the Department of Alcohol and Drug Programs, and the Office of Criminal Justice Planning, as well as the U.S. State Department and the U.S. Bureau of Prisons. He is the author of *Heroin and Politicians: The Failure of Public Policy to Control Addiction in America* and he has published articles in research journals that include the *Journal of Addictive Diseases,* the *Journal of Alcohol & Drug Education,* and *Borderlands Studies.*

Dr. Bellis has been elected twice as city councilman and mayor of Signal Hill, California. He is credited with reforming the city's government, which was beset with allegations of police misuse of force, felony conflict of interest on the city council, and election fraud. He was featured on ABC's *20/20* in relation to his reform movement in Signal Hill.

He is also an accomplished saxophone and clarinet player. As a professional musician in the 1960s, he played with Jan and Dean, Dick Dale, and the Del-Tones, and had his own jazz quintet. Dr. Bellis lives in Lake Arrowhead, California, with his wife Ann and son James.

# CONTENTS

# Preface

I cruise into the Hotel Ritz in Ciudad Victoria, capital of the state of Tamaulipas, Mexico, and sit down like a customer with five street-walking prostitutes on a worn couch. It is a steamy Wednesday afternoon in the summer of 1998. The sign out front reads "Hotel Ritz," but it is here, in a tiny street-front brothel near the city's main public market, that these female sex workers (FSWs) have sex with customers. You can buy anything in the market, for instance, opium, in the old days. The Hotel Ritz's front desk is used for renting out the sex servers' rooms at 5 pesos each (about 75 cents at the 1998 exchange rate).

Some of the women are dressed in tight-fitting miniskirts. Others wear jeans or regular dresses. They are eighteen to forty-five years old, ranging from slim to plump, beautiful to homely. The women are clean, well-groomed, and they smell good. I give each of them my university business card, quietly explaining that I am not there for sex. I tell them I am a California State University professor studying the relationships between commercial sex work, injected drug use, and AIDS. I say that I have interviewed many Southern California prostitutes, want twenty minutes of their time for short interviews, and will pay each of them 35 pesos ($5 at the time) for answering forty-eight questions about their lives as prostitutes and how they feel about AIDS and drugs. With that, I individually interview ten sex workers at the Hotel Ritz.

An old woman off the "reception" area inspects a man's penis for signs of sexually transmitted diseases (STDs). Her customary tip: 5 pesos. (For years, it had been routine for sex servers to examine potential customers for a chancre—the primary sore of syphilis which is healed in three to five weeks—or for a discharge which would be a sign of gonorrhea.) A twenty-minute sex act with one of the ten prostitutes working the Hotel Ritz—usually straight intercourse, sometimes "half-and-half"—is 35 pesos. One can get a couple of hours for 70 pesos. All of the FSWs who use the Hotel Ritz make sure that customers wear condoms.

Each FSW leads me back to her room for the interview. Their rooms are small, clean, each with a bed and sheet, bare lightbulb, small nightstand, maybe a mirror, and an omnipresent toilet paper roll.

They are very cooperative, interested in my research, and answer not-so-subtle questions such as, "What kind of sex do most of your clients want?", "Do you perform anal sex?" (*"Lo haces por el culo?"*), "Do you give head?" (*"Te parece bien por la boca, chupa la verga?"*), "Do you inspect or wash off your customer's penis?", or "How many prostitutes around here work unregistered?" (*"Cuantas mujeres alrededor de este barrio trabajan sin boleto?"*).

This book is about so-called streetwalkers such as these, their drug and sexual practices, and the relationship of such risky behavior to HIV (human immunodeficiency virus) and hepatitis C virus (HCV) infections. The data are drawn from a comparison of San Bernardino, California, female street sex workers (hereafter, FSWs) with their FSW counterparts in Mexico.

The differences between the Mexican and American FSWs were startling. The Mexicans were *choir girls* compared to their beaten up, sick, toothless, heroin-addicted Southern California sisters. Many more of the Americans had been through the drug/jail/john wringer compared with the Mexicans. This book summarizes those differences and sheds light on new directions for U.S. prostitution and heroin-control policies. These laws are currently so interwoven that they reinforce each other and account for a deadly circle of crime and disease, including AIDS, and now, hepatitis C.

By the time I got to Ciudad Victoria, I had already interviewed seventy-two San Bernardino street prostitutes. Later, I surveyed 102 FSWs in Tijuana, Baja California, Ciudad Juárez, Chihuahua, Ciudad Victoria, Tamaulipas, and Cuernavaca, Morelos. The American and Mexican FSWs were compared in multiple categories: drug use; sexual and health practices; and criminal histories. I wanted to uncover the relationship of these risk behaviors to infection with HIV, the etiological agent of acquired immunodeficiency syndrome (AIDS), and other STDs such as the rapidly spreading hepatitis C (HCV) virus.

A plethora of research has been conducted associating IDU (intravenous drug use), prostitution, and AIDS. Why *another* book on commercial sex, injected drug use, and AIDS? I wrote this book with four motivations in mind.

(1) *My heroin addiction.* Long before becoming a professor I was a heroin addict. I kicked the heroin habit approximately 200 times. This experience showed me the drug's effects, addiction treatment and rehabilitation, and addict street life, such as dealing drugs and seeing women prostitute for drug money. I have ingested almost every drug in the book—heroin and opium, methadone, LSD, PCP (phencyclidine; "angel dust"), peyote, psilocybin, weed, cocaine, amphetamines, methamphetamines, barbiturates ("fender-benders," "knee walkers"), and almost every other mind-altering substance known. Addiction is not confined to one substance (e.g., "polydrug abuse").

With this background, when the AIDS scare hit in the early 1980s, my curiosity piqued: I wondered if Southern California street prostitutes, hooking for drug money, were afraid of AIDS. Did their knowledge and fear of AIDS prompt any changes in their at-risk behavior, such as less sharing of injection paraphernalia and not having sex with multiple partners without condoms? I proposed to find out, and interviewed seventy-two street FSWs in San Bernardino, California in 1988.

(2) *Narcotic addiction treatment program experience.* Serving in several positions including directorships, board memberships, and counselorships between 1970 and 1985, I obtained millions of dollars in federal and state addiction treatment grants for thirty-five different addiction treatment and rehabilitation programs in the Los Angeles area.

In these programs I interviewed about 10,000 addicts in different treatment modalities: inpatient and outpatient detoxification using short-term methadone therapy; residential therapeutic communities of the Synanon variety; drug-free counseling programs; and Southern California's original methadone maintenance clinics. This was before the "privatization" of narcotic addiction treatment. In the early 1970s, I trained some of the biggest methadone maintenance program "entrepreneurs" in the United States. Now, they each own strings of twenty to thirty methadone clinics, even in Mexico, with up to 700 clients in each.

Most of the addiction treatment programs I managed and evaluated were in Boyle Heights, a quintessential Mexican barrio just east of downtown Los Angeles on the left bank of the Los Angeles River, and in south Ontario, California—both predominantly Hispanic barrios. One program, the Narcotics Prevention Project (NPP), was the first of its kind in Los Angeles's near East Side, a gang area with more addicts per square mile than perhaps anywhere in the city, and maybe on Earth. In the early 1970s, I wrote grants for NPP and the West End Drug Abuse Control Project in Ontario that funded the first treatment slots for heroin addicts in these areas.

NPP was started by Latino inmates released back to the community in 1967 from the California State Correctional Facility at Susanville. I began at NPP as an intake worker, graduated to "grant writer/ program evaluator," and ended up as vice chair of their board of directors. Thus, I saw this program from three levels: first as the strung-out client, then as a staffer, and then as a board member.

As a treatment program staffer, I encountered many female addicts who financed their heroin habits through prostitution. Clients such as "Rosie" from Chino, a big, tall, handsome, blond woman in her mid-twenties. She was always in and out of jail on drug and prostitution convictions. She would detox in my program to beat court cases, then always relapse to heroin using prostitution to finance her habit which would again grow to such proportions that she would return to detox six months later. Round and round Rosie spun on this addict-prostitute wheel. These women had no "pimps" in the usual sense (men living off the earnings of sex workers). Some had drug-addicted boy-friends who would shoot-up their profits, sometimes scoring dope for them. For these women, Aid to Families with Dependent Children (AFDC) paid the rent and utilities, Medi-Cal covered health insurance, food stamps fed them, while street prostitution fed their voracious heroin habits. (No such social welfare "safety net" exists for Mexican prostitutes.)

The prostitutes I treated were always getting robbed, raped, beaten up, and sometimes murdered by crazy johns in their interminable pursuit of heroin money. Because of my familiarity with these women, I could relate to them, talk their language, and understand the antecedents of their drug and family problems. I could go into the streets and easily interview them, anytime, anywhere. Thus, as an addiction treatment professional for thirty-two years, I have a deep interest in the relationship between commercial sex work, addiction, and by 1985, the growing AIDS epidemic that prompted this book.

(3) *Fluency in Spanish.* I speak fluent Spanish, which enabled me to get the information I needed for this book from Mexican sex work-

ers and government officials. My upbringing among Latinos in Los Angeles, my Spanish language education in both high school and college, and my experience while living and working as a musician in Mexico in the 1960s has given me the language skills I needed to gather data.

(4) *Experience as a Public Servant.* In the 1980s, I was a city councilman and mayor of Signal Hill, California, where I reformed a corrupt municipal administration, including its police department. Pacific Coast Highway (U.S. 101) etches the boundary between Signal Hill and Long Beach. Street prostitutes openly worked this stretch of interstate urban highway. Most were heroin addicts in search of money for a fix. I routinely fielded complaints about them:

> Mayor Bellis, my sister-in-law [visiting] here from Kansas, just got hit on three times by johns while she was walking to the 7-Eleven for a gallon of milk. I want you to *do* something about those whores working down on Coast Highway and all their tricks.

Local business owners and neighborhood organizations also complained that streetwalkers hurt their operations. Constituent service demanded that I call my new reform-minded chief of police. This translated into arresting the women for soliciting, being under the influence and possession of heroin, or pushing them somewhere else, mainly into neighboring Long Beach. Since their arrest charges routinely ran to being under the influence of heroin, I knew most of the women were addicts. I always wondered, around 1983 and 1984, as AIDS began receiving a barrage of news coverage, if these women were scared of the disease and whether this drove them to be more cautious in their sexual and drug-using behavior.

After my appointment as professor of public administration at California State University, San Bernardino, in 1985, I decided to interview some San Bernardino heroin-addicted female street sex workers to find out how they were reacting to the AIDS epidemic. Were they sharing narcotic-injection "outfits" less or making customers wear condoms for protection?

In 1988, I interviewed seventy-two heroin-addicted FSWs in San Bernardino. Then I interviewed a total of 102 Mexican street prostitutes (Table 1). Twenty-six of them were interviewed in June, 1996 on the streets of Tijuana, Baja California Norte. I then surveyed sev-

TABLE 1. Mexican Interview Sites and Sample Sizes

| | |
|---|---|
| Tijuana | *n* = 26 |
| Ciudad Juárez | *n* = 27 |
| Ciudad Victoria | *n* = 27 |
| Cuernavaca | *n* = 22 |
| TOTAL *n* = 102 Mexican Street FSWs | |

enty-six more Mexican sex workers during April and May, 1998 in Ciudad Juárez, Chihuahua, Ciudad Victoria, Tamaulipas, and Cuernavaca, Morelos.

I questioned whether these Mexican women differed from the American FSWs according to sociodemographic factors such as age, education, children, marital status, drug use, duration of sex work, condom use, criminality, and knowledge and fear of AIDS. Answers to these questions might help to inform the context of public policy-making in the United States and Mexico to more rationally control heroin, prostitution, and HIV/ STDs.

## Plan of This Book

The Introduction sketches the theoretical context, research questions, and the relationship between AIDS, intravenous drug use, and sex work. Chapter 2 follows the spread of HIV through drug injection and prostitution. It summarizes the incidence, prevalence, and modes of infection in reported AIDS cases among U.S. and Mexican FSWs. Chapter 3 is a short history of heroin, prostitution, and their relationship. Chapter 4 describes the Mexican study setting, methods, and subjects. Chapter 5 presents and analyzes the comparative findings from the Mexican and Southern California studies. Chapter 6 suggests policy changes to reduce AIDS and other STDs among Mexican and American prostitutes, and asks: Where do we go from here and how do we get there?

# Chapter 1

# Introduction

Jesus said to [the chief priests and elders] . . . the prostitutes are entering the kingdom of God before you.

Matthew 21:31
*The Living New Testament* (1967)

Prostitution and mind-altering drug use have been common threads in the social fabric of humanity. Commercial sex work has existed throughout recorded history, from biblical writings to the respected *hetaerae,* or concubines, of ancient Greece. At almost no time in any civilized society has sex for hire not been commonplace—while at the same time, those who have legislated against it and those who have paid lip service to the legislation, have, in large numbers, employed the services of the very sex workers they condemned. The politicians' records are pretty clear: skewer these people, while sipping tea, little finger in the air.

For thousands of years, people have also taken drugs to alter their moods, relax, feel better, feel different, escape, and avoid pain. This has eventuated in an increasing demand for a variety of psychoactive substances. Opium (Greek: *opion,* poppy juice) is obtained by incising the unripe seed pod of the poppy *(Papaver somniferum).* Sumerians in what is now southern Iraq around 7000 B.C. told of its power to produce a sense of delight or satisfaction. Opium was among the most common drugs of the Assyrians and the ancient Egyptians. In Europe, opium poppies were found in Hungary around 1200 B.C., and traces of their cultivation have been uncovered near ancient lake dwellings in Switzerland. Of all the opiates, heroin—so named for its heroic pain-relieving properties—has received the most attention.

The time is long past due to turn the cards face up on America's and Mexico's street sex industries, and their relationship to IDU and

*1*

the spread of AIDS. This book is about the differences in AIDS knowledge, fear of AIDS, health, sex, criminal histories, and injected drug use practices that I discovered among seventy-two San Bernardino, California, hard-core FSWs and 102 of their counterparts in four big Mexican cities. My first Mexican interviews were conducted in June 1996 when I surveyed twenty-six borderland female street sex workers on the streets of Tijuana, Baja California Norte (Bellis, 1999; 2001). During the summer of 1998, I conducted seventy-six more interviews: twenty-seven in Ciudad Juárez, Chihuahua; twenty-seven in Ciudad Victoria, Tamaulipas; and twenty-two in Cuernavaca, Morelos (Bellis, 2001). To confirm my Mexican results, I interviewed ten additional street FSWs in Tijuana in June, 1999. The results were exactly the same.

My wife and fourteen-year-old son accompanied me on the 1998 Mexican prostitution research trip; we drove around fourteen Mexican states in a small R.V. My family's understanding was complete as I searched out prostitutes to interview in their customary hooking locales, mainly on the streets and in small, street-front brothels. I felt that street-level FSWs, because they occupy the bottom rung of the commercial sex work ladder, would be more likely than "high class" sex workers to be intravenous drug users and to spread HIV. I questioned whether the fear of contracting AIDS was scaring any of these American and Mexican women into being more careful with drug injection, their customers, other risk behaviors, and health checkups. How do the two groups stack up against each other? How do Mexican laws compare with the American approach to prostitution?

## THEORY, RESEARCH DESIGN, AND STUDY LIMITATIONS

### Theoretical Context

Science is the search for causes; it assumes that *everything* has a cause. There are many reasons why Mexican street prostitutes are a lot better off (have less HIV risk exposure) than their Southern California counterparts. The search for explanations, however, is like staring down into a plate of spaghetti: every strand is entangled with every other. Sorting things out can be difficult.

Propositions as to why American FSWs are more at-risk for HIV transmission than their Mexican cousins are intertwined with multiple theoretical constructs and hypotheses. Following are a few:

## *Political Science/Politics/Public Policy Hypotheses*

H1: The Mexican prostitution regulation system requires STD testing and health surveillance of prostitutes. It is thus more effective at stopping AIDS among FSWs than America's punitive, criminal approach to prostitution.

H2: Mexican social services policy provides no "safety net" for the poor; they have to work. For prostitutes, they must keep their noses to the grindstone; it is their "job," they have no time or money to mess around with drugs. In contrast, the United States still has a public welfare system that provides such a safety net, allowing street prostitutes to live off direct welfare grants (*and* food stamps, *and* Medicaid, *and* housing allowances) while pocketing their prostitution money for dope.

H3: Politicians seek votes. American elected officials are more likely to come down hard on prostitution and drugs than are Mexican politicians, where drugs and prostitution are not as important in the minds of voters. This puts American FSWs in a more risky AIDS infection position than Mexican FSWs.

## *Sociological Theory*

H1: Mexican prostitutes are too poor to afford drugs, and thus are at less risk for HIV transmission through unsterile drug injection equipment.

H2: Illicit drug misuse is more taboo among Mexican than American women, so Mexican women (and Mexican FSWs) are less likely to abuse drugs than American FSWs. The same holds true among Mexican versus U.S. males.

H3: Compared with their "hip" urban-bred American counterparts, Mexican FSWs are mainly "country girls" who have come to the big city in search of fortune, and are thus more naive about drugs—especially injected heroin.

*Gender Theory*

> H1: Male dominance is one factor forcing females into prostitution. Men have more choices in society. This puts FSWs in the position of being more at risk for HIV transmission.

*Pharmacological/Substance Abuse Theory*

> H1: American prostitutes are more likely than Mexican FSWs to be narcotic addicts. Opioid addiction is characterized by tolerance and withdrawal. Addicts in acute stages of withdrawal will take extreme chances to relieve their narcotic craving ("yen"). They are thus more at risk for HIV infection than nonaddicts such as the Mexican FSWs.

*Economic Theory*

> H1: Economically, the price of heroin is "price inelastic." Addicts will crawl through the sewer and beg to buy, at *any* price. They thus are likely to take huge risks (prostitution; unprotected sex) to get the money for heroin, and use any means available to inject it quick, such as unsterile injection paraphernalia contaminated with HIV or hepatitis C virus.

> H2: Mexico is more of a drug-exporting than a drug-using country. Its main client is the United States. Heroin is more available on the streets of the United States than Mexico, so American FSWs are more likely to be addicts than are Mexican FSWs.

*Historical Theory*

> H1: Around the time of Prohibition in the United States (1919-1933), prostitution was made illegal and many bordellos were closed. This forced prostitutes into street-level prostitution, where they were less subject to regulation and control that might have led to better STD testing and surveillance. Prostitution is legal with health exams in most parts of Mexico.

*Criminal Justice Theory*

H1: Drug and prostitution criminalization gives police, courts, and the corrections system something to do. It is their raison d'être. It creates a kind of drug abuse/ prostitution "industrial complex" with its own congeries of powerful interest groups with built-in momentum to continue the criminal justice system of police, courts, and corrections. Mexico, too, has this, but to a much lesser extent than the United States.

*Moral and Religious Theories*

H1: Puritanism and Calvinism in America have contributed to the "moralistic" prohibition of drugs and prostitution, which has led to black markets, higher prices, and repressive laws against these behaviors. American prostitutes are thus more subject to criminal sanctions. Mexican Catholicism is more "tolerant" of prostitution; it provides sinners more "wiggle room." Repentance in the Catholic religion (most Mexicans are Catholic) generally takes place in the privacy of the confessional, where penance is tantamount to forgiveness. For prostitution, "zones of tolerance" exist in Mexican cities, where prostitution is legal and more closely regulated, leading to less drug abuse and STD transmission.

*Mass Communications Theory*

H1: American and Western European film, fiction books, and TV are more likely than Mexican media to depict opiate addiction and prostitution (*Panic in Needle Park, Trainspotting, Traffic, COPS,* and *Frontline* on TV, etc.).

These theories and more might explain the differences between Mexican and U.S. subjects.

## Research Design and Study Limitations

Research included FSWs in the United States and Mexico. San Bernardino field interviews were purposely restricted to IDUs, since

I assumed that they would be most at risk for HIV infection. Interview subjects in Tijuana, Ciudad Juárez, Ciudad Victoria, and Cuernavaca were picked randomly, with no distinction between FSWs who were IDUs and those who were not.

The research protocol for both the 1988 San Bernardino interviews and 1996-1999 Mexican street studies was straightforward. The data collection strategy involved developing a standardized, forty-eight-item, interviewer-administered, hybrid questionnaire (see the Appendix).

In San Bernardino, I first visited the police department's narcotics and vice detail and told them not to arrest me out on the streets for soliciting prostitutes; I was a university researcher not a "trick." A San Bernardino police officer who was a student of mine accompanied me on my first night of interviewing. He introduced me around to the initial FSWs I interviewed, and told them my purpose.

San Bernardino itself, a tough, working-class city of 200,000, sixty miles east of downtown Los Angeles, seemed like a good setting for sex-worker interviews. It is the county seat for a 20,164-square mile county, the largest in the contiguous United States, and bigger than the combined land masses of New Jersey, Massachusetts, Delaware, and Rhode Island. It has a blighted downtown, above-average unemployment, and higher-than-average crime (the 1988 homicide rate surpassed both that of Miami and Houston). In 2000, its county government was wracked by corruption scandals headlined in the *Los Angeles Times*—bribery, kickbacks, and extortion. Measured by total population, the county is the sixteenth largest in the United States. San Bernardino has suffered deeply from military base closures (Norton Air Force Base), urban flight, and failed economic revitalization policies. Over half of its population is on public assistance (Flanigan, 1998). In a nutshell, the city is in trouble and it has long been the destination for johns seeking to buy sex off the street.

I restricted my San Bernardino street prostitute interviews to those who were injecting heroin, and they were not hard to find. As I rapidly screened each sex worker for an interview, a visual check of them quickly confirmed signs of heroinism: constricted pupils, multiple intravenous puncture wounds in their arms or on the backs of their hands ("marks," "tracks"), and the somnolence characteristic of narcotic intoxication.

The questions I asked them included:

- Demographics
- Types of sexual behavior
- Types of clients and number serviced per day
- History of STDs and HIV infection
- Condom use and client attitudes toward condoms
- Alcohol and other drug dependence
- Criminal history
- Knowledge and attitudes about AIDS

Members of this purposive sample of heroin-addicted subjects were questioned in their own customary environment—mainly on the streets, but some in sleazy motel rooms, in my car, beside and even inside big rigs at a truck stop along the busy I-10 freeway. The old Truckadero truck stop was a bustling place. Prostitutes were hopping from truck sleeper to truck sleeper, receiving their directions from the drivers over CB radios. Truckers pulling in off the freeway were lining up "dates." I interviewed prostitutes there, and also witnessed numerous sales of stolen merchandise and immigrant smuggling.

During an interview in a cheap motel room, a respondent's two-year-son played with a broken, dirty, heroin-injecting syringe on the floor. My respondents spoke freely and with no reticence to questions such as, "Do you give butt (sodomy)?" ("Hell no," said most, "unless I'm paid a lot extra.")

My modus operandi in initiating street interviews was to cruise up in my Toyota to a possible subject, introduce myself, scope her out fast to see if she was an addict, and give her my university business card. This got their attention fast. What trick hands over his business card? It helped prove that I was not the police. I told each of the seventy-two women that I was a university professor at Cal State, San Bernardino, and a former heroin addict myself, out interviewing women like them to see how they felt about HIV/AIDS while working the streets and "shooting stuff." In field research like this, self-revelation by the researcher is useful in gaining respondent confidence (Madge, 1965). I asked each FSW if she would be willing to let me confidentially interview her, which would require about twenty minutes, for $20. I told them that I did not want names, that I was using anonymous statistics. Almost every woman approached in this fashion was extremely cooperative and open. Some respondents provided other subjects for interview. At one motel, they literally lined up to be interviewed and to get their $20. Afterward, I watched some head straight for the drug connection's "pad" to score more dope.

I found that though knowledgeable about and fearful of AIDS, these San Bernardino street FSWs had not changed their sexual or IDU behavior. They did little to protect themselves or their customers from HIV infection. They did *not* abstain from injecting heroin (and sometimes cocaine, or methamphetamine); they did *not* rely on disinfected and unshared injection equipment (syringes/needles, cookers [spoons or metal bottle caps], cottons, and rinse water); they did *not* require condom use; they had *not* undergone regular medical examinations and routine testing for HIV/STDs (Bellis, 1989; 1990).

The compulsive engine of heroin need and the inexorable drive for drug money compelled them to continue prostituting on the streets for drug money, ignoring AIDS risk. These personal interviews demonstrated that while the rational, logical side of a subject's brain knew about and was deathly afraid of AIDS because she shared "outfits" with other IDUs or because of sex acts with infected customers and addict boyfriends, the irrationality produced by narcotic addiction compelled risky behavior. Other studies have noted that prostitutes have a high level of HIV/AIDS knowledge, but continue to engage in unsafe sexual behavior (Smith, Lockett, and Bala, 1996).

Based on these interviews, I obtained a treatment grant from the State of California to provide free methadone maintenance for 100 such women in a private methadone maintenance clinic in San Bernardino. My follow-up study of that experimental program showed that free methadone significantly reduced their HIV-risk behavior, such as IDU and prostitution for drug money, thus lessening their HIV exposure (Bellis, 1993).

## *MEXICAN STUDY*

In the Mexican study, I conducted individual face-to-face FSW interviews on the streets of Tijuana during June 1996, and in the other Mexican cities from May-June 1998. These Mexican women were randomly interviewed. The same standardized, forty-eight-item questionnaire employed in the 1988 San Bernardino study was used with the Mexican FSWs.

In Tijuana and Ciudad Juárez, I approached women who obviously were sex workers in those cities' well-known *zonas* (red-light districts). Police in these two Mexican cities, perhaps because of the border locations and appeal to American johns, are less likely to force sex workers off the streets and into brothels. The FSWs at the bottom of the prostitution ladder in Ciudad Victoria and Cuernavaca are confined by local regulations to cheap, working-class *cantinas,* and small hotels *(hotelitos)* such as the Hotel Ritz in Ciudad Victoria, a brothel despite its upper class name.

### Small Sample Sizes

The comparative U.S. and Mexican results may be criticized from three directions. First, the small samples may not typify all street FSWs in the cities studied, nor in the United States or Mexico. Larger samples could have yielded more statistical significance. Nonetheless, the size of the Mexican samples has significance for the locales in which they were drawn. For example, in Tijuana I counted roughly 300 FSWs on one square block of this city's *zona roja* around 10 p.m. on a Friday night in June 1996. My sample of twenty-six was just under 10 percent of the women I counted working this central area of Tijuana's famous downtown prostitution *zona.*

The seventy-two-member San Bernardino sample, based on my own field observations and interviews with San Bernardino police, seemed typical of street FSWs in that city.

### Comparability of the San Bernardino and Mexican Samples

Second, the Mexican and San Bernardino samples are not strictly comparable. My research protocol for the San Bernardino study specified interviewing IDUs only. This was to ensure that I surveyed FSWs most at risk for HIV transmission. I only interviewed San Bernardino FSWs who were injecting heroin, and they were not hard to find. Nine out of ten FSWs who were approached as possible subjects for my street survey were under the influence of narcotics, mainly black tar heroin.

Put simply, in terms of time frame, things have not changed much. By 2001, a San Bernardino Police Department narcotics and vice officer told the press that "I have not met a prostitute [in San Bernardino] who does not use narcotics" (Martinez, personal interview, 2001). On the other hand, the Tijuana, Ciudad Juárez, Ciudad Victoria, and Cuernavaca subjects were not restricted to IDUs; I picked them at random on the streets, or in brothels or *cantinas*. The Mexican and San Bernardino samples might be said to be comparing "apples and oranges"—San Bernardino FSWs chosen specifically because they were IDUs versus a purposive sample of Mexican FSWs *not* screened for IDU. However, almost all of the women I randomly approached in San Bernardino were under the influence of injected drugs; it was hard to find some who were not. "Typical" San Bernardino FSWs were heroin addicts; "typical" FSWs in Mexico were *not* IDUs. So, the U.S. and Mexican data have limitations along the IDU comparability factor, but, nonetheless, allow for drawing some tentative parallels regarding HIV-risk behavior between average San Bernardino and Mexican street FSWs.

### Changes in FSW Drug Use Patterns in San Bernardino Since the 1988 Interviews

Third, my San Bernardino interviews were conducted in 1988. Have drug-use patterns changed in the intervening time period? Since then, have there been any significant HIV-risk behavior changes among this population, such as less IDU or more condom use and medical checkups? These factors affect HIV seropositivity rates among street sex workers, but questions about current drugs of choice among Southern California FSWs cannot be answered definitively because local and national drug use trend data are either not always available or are contradictory.

Assessing the changing scope of drug-use patterns among street FSWs is difficult. No consensus exists on what the patterns are at any given time or over time. Surveys have been incapable of measuring these changes nationwide because data at the local level are inadequate. Few systematic data are routinely collected on FSW drug use patterns at city and county levels, with the exception of a few information systems. Generally, intermittent surveys are relied on for assessing the scope and range of FSW drug-use patterns.

Although data have not yet been gathered, and few estimates are available, five factors seemed to account for the general changes in drug-use patterns among this population. A major source of variation is found in the complex relationship between:

- Drug "era"
- Illicit drug costs and availability
- FSW race/ethnicity
- FSW position on the sex worker hierarchy
- Geographic location of sex workers

The 1988 street survey of San Bernardino FSWs determined that they were heroin addicts. What about FSWs working the streets now?

To update the San Bernardino findings compared with those obtained in Mexico, in 1999 I interviewed fifteen vice and narcotic police officers representing ten different Southern California law enforcement agencies, including two undercover operators from the San Bernardino Police Department. They were drawn from:

- Los Angeles County Sheriff's Department
- Riverside County Sheriff's Department
- San Bernardino County Sheriff's Department
- San Bernardino Police Department
- Ontario Police Department (San Bernardino County)
- Upland Police Department (San Bernardino County)
- Indio Police Department (Riverside County)
- Garden Grove Police Department (Orange County)
- Fullerton Police Department (Orange County)
- Los Angeles Police Department

These departments range from the 11,000-officer LAPD and 11,000-deputy Los Angeles County Sheriff's Department, and 3,000-strong San Bernardino County Sheriff's Department, to smaller agencies such as the Indio and Garden Grove Police Departments. I asked each respondent four questions after telling them about my 1988 San Bernardino FSW heroin use findings:

- What are the main drugs of abuse you *currently* (1999 versus 1988) find among street FSWs, and how are they ingested?
- Are street FSWs any more careful than they were ten years ago about requiring condom use?

- Are IDU street FSWs more or less likely than they were ten years ago to share drug injection paraphernalia?
- Have your agency's prostitution abatement programs been successful or not in suppressing street prostitution?

Interviews with a cross section of commanders, patrol, and undercover vice and narcotics officers from these departments updated my picture of current HIV-risk behavior among street FSWs in the Southern California megalopolis. The portrait is complex and ever-changing. Following are some of the significant findings.

## MAIN DRUGS OF ABUSE AND INJECTION METHODS

The general notion that IDU is fading must be taken with a grain of salt. Conversations with police officers over the past ten years and my own observations indicate that most low-level female sex workers still go back and forth between heroin and other drugs (Farmer, personal interview, 1999).

The fifteen Southern California police officers who I interviewed, and who regularly interact with street FSWs, report that they tend to find pipes for smoking meth or crack in the FSWs' purses. In contrast, ten years ago, they found syringes for injecting heroin. This suggests an increase in crack cocaine (called crack because it "crackles" in the cooking process) and methamphetamine smoking and a decrease in injecting heroin. The type of "meth" most prevalent on the streets, since it is the cheapest and most easily produced variety, is amphetamine sulfate. Amphetamine hydrochloride ("crystal meth," "ice") is more expensive, trendier with the Hollywood set, and less prevalent among FSWs. As two San Bernardino Police Department undercover vice detectives reported during a personal interview with me in 1999,

> Sixty percent of them [street FSWs] today are smoking meth. When we bust 'em we find pipes, not outfits [for heroin injection] in their purses. Back in the late 80s, heroin was big. But recently, heroin's down. Except among the Mexican hookers; they're more into shooting heroin. But 85 percent to 90 percent of the prostitutes we bust in our operations are on meth or smoke rock [cocaine]. But, again, it all depends on where they're from, who they are. Blacks are more into smoking crack, whites

smoke or shoot meth, and Mexican hookers are more into heroin. But, you know, it all depends on what's cheap right now and on the streets. Heroin'll be back. It seems like these women don't care what they use; it's what's available. (personal communication)

In some populations, patterns may emerge from geographic location, and the cost and availability of drugs on the street. In others, drug-use patterns may be more related to the ethnic or racial origin of FSWs and their "neighborhood." Like San Bernardino, San Diego is known as one of the meth capitals of the United States. There, more than 40 percent of the criminal defendants have methamphetamine in their systems at arrest ("Injunction Best Tack," 2001).

What combination of these factors primarily accounts for drug use patterns is not clear, but some preliminary conclusions can be made. For example, street FSWs working in Southern California are primarily from lower-class, slum, ghetto, barrio, or working-class communities. Smoking crack cocaine is especially widespread among African-American street FSWs.

A detective with the organized crime unit of the Los Angeles Police Department told me that in her experience, "Most streetwalkers smoke crack and marijuana. Others inject methamphetamine. We aren't seeing many heroin users" (personal communication, 1999).

Smoking and injecting methamphetamine (a powerful central nervous system stimulant whose long-term effects include liver damage, stroke, and death) are more prevalent among white FSWs. Hispanic street FSWs have strong links to the neighborhood, or barrio where heroin traditionally (because of connections to Mexico) is more readily available, and, thus, are more likely to use heroin. The prevalent types of heroin among these women are Mexican black tar *(goma)* and "Mexican Brown" powdered heroin. Black tar sells for about $25 a quarter gram, Mexican Brown around $100 a quarter gram. Because of its impurities, the tar heroin causes serious infections at injection sites and cannot be used over sustained periods of time without producing local necrosis and bone exposure.

The city of Indio, about fifteen minutes from ritzy Palm Desert, California, home to many of the low-paid workers who manicure golf courses and who are maids and kitchen help in the Palm Springs area resort industry, is primarily Hispanic. So is Coachella, its next-door neighbor. The upscale community of Indian Wells wanted to pay

Coachella to take its low-income housing allotment. Heroin use among street FSWs is especially widespread in Indio and Coachella, with an estimated use rate of 80 percent. A vice sergeant in Indio told me in 1999 that,

> In Indio we work lots of stings with undercover officers posing as johns and reverse-stings with our operators posing as prostitutes. It's mainly heroin use among street FSWs in Indio and next door in Coachella. They're injecting Mexican black tar heroin. There's lots of it around. We're only an hour from Mexico. These towns are 80 percent Hispanic, and drug use among prostitutes around here seems to vary by ethnic group. The Hispanics use heroin, blacks crack cocaine, and whites use meth. You'll find the higher class call girls and escort service prostitutes up in Palm Springs [fifteen miles away] don't tend to use heroin. They're either not into drugs that heavy or those that use, smoke speed [methamphetamine]. (personal interview)

A twenty-three-year veteran corporal who books prostitutes at the Riverside County Jail in Indio confirmed that,

> Most all the women prostitutes we get in here from Indio and Coachella are shooting heroin. It's so cheap and available around here, close to Mexico. It's about $10 a quarter gram. Mexican black tar heroin. Most of our prostitutes are Hispanics. The few Anglo prostitutes we get mainly smoke meth, and the African Americans tend to smoke crack. (personal interview)

So in Indio and Coachella, heroin use seems to be linked to FSW ethnicity and geographic locale.

In addition to ethnicity and neighborhood, another way of viewing drug-use patterns among street FSWs in Southern California is along the continuum of underlying, cyclical heroin use. A Hispanic detective on the Ontario, California Police Department told me in 1999 that,

> Street hookers I interview mostly smoke meth and crack. The high is more intense than heroin. Meth and crack here are cheaper and more available than heroin. I don't see or hear of more heroin on the streets over the last two years. *But I think heroin will get popular again among street prostitutes. That's*

*the way it goes; it's cyclical.* [emphasis mine] (personal interview)

Observations of FSWs' drug-use patterns of any given period tend to relate the drugs of choice to those of the particular ethnic groups prominent in the urban lower class during that period.

Illicit drug-use patterns among street FSWs are cyclical over time. The last thirty years in Southern California show four distinct periods. During the 1960s, the persistent drugs of abuse among street FSWs were marijuana, Benzedrine, heroin, and LSD. Through the 1970s until the mid-1980s, heroin was the primary drug. By the late 1980s and early 1990s, smokeable crack cocaine and methamphetamines began to dominate the street drug scene and use by FSWs. Use of these drugs was fueled by their cheaper cost compared with heroin, their ability to be smoked rather than injected, and their wide availability on the streets.

There is little hard evidence to support the notion that the crack/meth trend is permanent. Much remains to be learned about the relationship between IDU and factors such as drug cost/availability, ethnicity, location, changing urban economy, and changing neighborhood dynamics.

## *CONCERN OF STREET FSWs IN REQUIRING CONDOM USE COMPARED TO TEN YEARS AGO*

Currently, street FSWs seem more insistent on condom use than they were in 1988. Addiction and HIV prevention education may have altered their risky behavior, such as requiring more customers to use condoms, or not sharing heroin injection paraphernalia. Certainly, street-level HIV prevention/education programs among addicts, such as those conducted by Inland AIDS Project in Riverside, California, which borders San Bernardino, have intensified in the past ten years. If the 1988 interviews were replicated now, the answers might be somewhat different.

Are police crackdowns on prostitutes having any effect? What seems to have changed the most in San Bernardino and other traditional street prostitution locales in U.S. cities, is the visibility and presence of FSWs on the streets. Many have disappeared from their old haunts, making it hard to find any of them to interview. Why, and, where, have they gone?

Street prostitutes are having less success evading the law. More intense police pressure beginning in the 1970s probably caused the proliferation of massage parlors in that decade, where soliciting is conducted inside. Suddenly, prostitutes became "masseuses." Cities and counties have tried to catch up by passing strict ordinances regulating massage parlors and the women who work there, but law enforcement resources are often committed to higher priority crimes. Police, pressured by legislators, local residents, and businesspersons, have forced prostitutes (and street drug dealers) to change their tactics. In one year, two undercover cops in San Bernardino arrested 280 street FSWs and johns (personal interview with two San Bernardino undercover narcotics detectives, 1999).

Streetwalkers are often judged to be a "public nuisance." They have been accused of flashing their breasts at motorists, urinating and defecating on private property, using drugs and alcohol, making threats, and bothering residents and the customers of area businesses.

By 1999, local San Bernardino plainclothes police officers had a permanent judicial injunction to use against prostitutes. The new, permanent court injunction in San Bernardino cited a list of thirty-six FSWs, including two who had since died of AIDS-related complications. By court order, these women were prohibited from a long list of specific behaviors, such as waving at cars or standing on private property. If they were caught doing anything prohibited in the order they could be jailed for contempt of court. "The beauty of the injunction," said Dwight Moore, supervising San Bernardino County deputy district attorney, "is that they don't have to be hooking. If they are walking where they were ordered not to, they can be arrested, making it a whole lot easier to clear the streets" (Martinez, 2001, p. A1).

An employee of a pawn shop in the area most frequented by street FSWs in the past said, "they would stand out in front of the store and harass customers. . . . Not anymore" (Fitzsimmons, 1999, p. B3). By 2001, a San Bernardino store owner said, "Before, it was a horrible problem. We had prostitutes 24 hours a day. It took a lot of work to get it into place, but it's worked very, very well. The injunction was successful in clearing the women off the streets either through arrests or by convincing them that certain areas did not welcome their services. The local newspaper cheered that this was "an outcome we feel very confident [about]." ("Injunction Best Tack," 2001, p. B7).

Customers are less willing to shop for sex along such streets subject to injunctions or which are routinely staked out by police doing stings (police as customers) and reverse stings (police as prostitutes). Anyone who has seen the television show *COPS* knows that undercover police change the officers for stings because the FSWs quickly learn to recognize them. It is not so critical to change female officers in reverse stings, since there are so many tricks that the women cannot be recognized anyway.

Johns have their cars impounded in Portland, Oakland, and San Diego, and their pictures and names are placed in newspapers in other cities. The theory is that if wives, friends, and employers see this, it will act as a deterrent. In California, the law allows judges to suspend for up to thirty days the driver's license of anyone convicted of soliciting a prostitute within 1,000 feet of a home and involving the use of a car.

The personal downside of this intense pressure on street sex workers is that they are being incarcerated for nonviolent drug and prostitution offenses and, as a result, leave behind their children who many times end up with unsuitable relatives or are bounced around in foster care. One can question whether they are really a threat to society. It seems that they just do not have the insurance, money, education, or support needed to turn their drug use around, so now they are "criminals."

Because of intense police busts of open-air drug markets and streetwalking, working FSWs have been exercising more discretion. Prostitution is no less prevalent; it is just that prostitutes, like drug dealers, have learned to move their trade *indoors*.

This has been greatly facilitated by the use of cell phones and pagers. For $30 a month, a customer and sex worker can have both a beeper and a cell phone. Scrambled strips of beeper numbers used in sex transactions make it hard for police to figure out the transactions should pagers get seized. Even the Internet is coming into play (Roane, 1998), and former streetwalkers are operating out of escort services listed in the yellow pages of city telephone books. Commercial, street-level sex workers have created a new technological connection with their customers without being exposed to the eyes of watching police, residents, and businesspeople. The days of buying sex straight off the street are rapidly disappearing, at least in Southern

Californian cities. The retreat from traditional street prostitution is attributed to a simple interrelationship: the commercial sex workers do
not want to get caught by police, and the available technology of
phones and pagers. The prostitutes have insulated themselves.

Prostitution is mainly arranged by phone now, "call and ball." Sex
workers build client lists so that they can arrange work by phone, not
on the street. It works like this: customers—"johns"—page the sex
worker who calls back and sets up the meet—it could be at a bus stop,
grocery store, post office, at the prostitute's motel room, or in the customer's bedroom. The transition from open-street prostitution has
forced the trade indoors where it is thriving. Sex is being sold just as
regularly, but not as blatantly. The changing street prostitution scene
is having an effect along many highways and byways—sweeping out
the "unsavory" open street prostitution. I experienced this in the
1980s when, as mayor of Signal Hill, California, I ordered police
sweeps of prostitutes adjacent to Pacific Coast Highway (U.S. 101).
The goal was to push them into Long Beach, whose border lay across
the street.

Until police develop a strategy to beat this new, higher technology
pattern, commercial sex workers will be on top of this cat-and-mouse
game. Another result of new technology is that those who conduct research among street FSWs have more difficulty finding them. Most
interview studies are conducted with sex workers in custody. These
subjects, however, tend to give different responses from those on the
streets. They are more remorseful, and usually not under the influence of drugs.

# Chapter 2

# Etiology of HIV Transmission

By now, almost everybody knows that AIDS is a blood-borne and sexually transmitted disease. HIV invades the body and damages its immune system (which protects the body from infections) and allows other "opportunistic" infectious agents to cause severe disease (CDC, 1988; Piot et al., 1988) such as *Pneumocystis carinii* pneumonia and lymphoma in the brain. (A minor infection such as pharyngitis can blossom into an overwhelming lethal disease.) AIDS-related complex (ARC) includes *Pneumocystis carniii,* a pulmonary manifestation, and Kaposi's sarcoma, a dermatologic malignancy involving deeper areas. Indeed, these conditions may be the first indicators of AIDS.

HIV-positive individuals ("seropositive") are those who have been infected with the AIDS virus, have developed antibodies to it, and may have the virus in the blood, but may not have the disease. Many positive reactors are asymptomatic. The following ad appeared in the personal column of a popular magazine: "GBM, 31, seeks intelligent, lit, and fun-loving GM, 25-40 for friendship, correspondence or more. *I'm pos. but healthy*" (*The Nation,* 1988, p. 34).

After six years, about a third of those infected with HIV develop clinical AIDS (Stevens et al., 1986). Some physicians predict that all who develop AIDS will die of the disease (Booth, 1988b; CDC, 1987c), though other researchers dispute this assertion. HIV antibodies are detectable by enzyme-linked immunosorbent assay (ELISA) and confirmed for a greater margin of certainty by a testing method called Western Blot. Heroin addicts who are HIVpositive can infect others through sharing narcotic injection paraphernalia and engaging in unprotected sex (Koop, 1986). AIDS is one of several infections transmitted by sexual contact. Others are gonorrhea, syphilis, genital herpes, chlamydia, chancroid, and granuloma inguinale, which are called venereal diseases.

HIV can be passed from infected men to normal women and from infected women to normal men through penis-vaginal intercourse (Koop, 1986) and fellatio when gum fissures and ulcerations exist (Wallace et al., 1996). It can be transmitted from infected men to other men, principally through anal intercourse. This is why sodomy is a major HIV risk factor for HIV acquisition in men who have sex with men. Sexual practices which cause small, often invisible, tears in the mucosa of the vagina, rectum, or penis are linked to HIV transmission. Other infections already present in the penis, rectum, vagina, or cervix facilitate transmission of HIV because direct access to the blood is gained.

HIV is transmitted by blood-to-blood contact between seropositive persons and normal individuals in four ways: (1) unprotected sexual contact (Koop, 1986); (2) transfusions with infected blood (CDC, 1987b); (3) perinatally from mother to neonate (Cowan et. al., 1984); and (4) sharing syringes and hypodermic needles or other skin penetrating instruments (Von Reyn, Fordham, and Mann, 1987). Blood, semen, and cervicovaginal fluid are the most potent agents of HIV transmission (Curran et al., 1988; Los Angeles County Department of Health Services, 1987; Vogt et al., 1986). The major risk factor for HIV infection in U.S. FSWs appears to be IDU.

## *INCIDENCE AND PREVALENCE OF HIV/AIDS*

Since the first AIDS cases were reported in 1981, by 1995 over 20 million persons worldwide had been diagnosed with the disease (Caldwell and Caldwell, 1996). By 1999, the estimated number of HIVpositive people worldwide was 30 million, including 1.5 million under age fifteen (Read, 1999). The number of people infected with HIV/AIDS is growing rapidly in less developed nations in Africa and in places such as India (Geeta, Lindan, and Hudes, 1995), the world's second most populous nation (Govindaraj, Govindaraj, and Appachu, 1998). Over 4 million South Africans—out of a population of 43 million—are HIV positive. Without dramatic interventions, 10 million South Africans will be HIV positive in less than ten years, and life expectancy for those under thirty-five will be cut in half (Herbert, 2001).

As of December 1997, 733,193 HIV/AIDS cases had been reported in the United States (Fleming et al., 1998; CDC, 2001). By

2002 the figure stood at 774,467, with 450,000 total deaths recorded (CDC, 2001; Cimons, 2001). Over one million Americans, roughly one in 2,500, reportedly (Root-Bernstein, 1996; Noll, 1996) are HIVpositive. Since 1993, however, the AIDS case rate/100,000 population has been declining, with a slight upturn noted in 2001.

By 1999, 2,503 AIDS cases had been reported in San Bernardino County, and a total of 500 in the city of San Bernardino. San Bernardino County ranks ninth among California's fifty-eight counties in AIDS cases (San Bernardino County, 2001).

The estimated number of deaths in the United States among persons reported with AIDS increased steadily through 1994, but since then, the number of deaths per 100,000 due to HIV/AIDS have declined among all racial/ethnic groups (Fleming et al., 1998; Dean-Gaitor, Fleming, and Ward, 1998; CDC, 2001; Maugh, 1998; San Bernardino County, 2001). AIDS has now fallen off the list of the top ten killers in the United States. AIDS deaths dropped for the first time in 1996 and the trend has continued. Although *death* from AIDS is declining steeply, the number of new HIV *infections* each year is essentially stable. In 1997, there were about 40,000 new infections, a number that remains steady. Significantly, among black males and females and Hispanics, the rate of new HIV infection is on the rise.

Is the AIDS epidemic under control? The incoming data are inconclusive. AIDS has dropped on the list of top causes of death. AIDS ranked as the fourteenth leading cause of death in the United States in 1997—down from eighth in 1996. These may be temporary and misleading signs.

The number of AIDS deaths decreased 44 percent in the United States during the first half of 1997. For that entire year, 16,865 died of opportunistic infections caused by AIDS, compared with 31,130 deaths in 1996. This is the lowest death rate level since 1987—the first year AIDS deaths were tracked.

Although there are fewer people dying from AIDS in the United States, more infections are still occurring. In 1999, there were an estimated 40,000 new HIV infections (Read, 1999). Los Angeles County is illustrative. There, reported cases of HIV/AIDS are still increasing: 3,169 total cases in 1996 versus 3,274 in 1997 (Los Angeles County Department of Health Services, 1997). Similar increases in new cases continued into 1999 and 2000 (Los Angeles County Department of Health Services, 1999b). In a four-month period in 1997, there were

159 new AIDS cases, compared with 192 in the same quarter of 1998 (Los Angeles County Department of Health Services, 1998a). By 1999, AIDS cases were still increasing (Los Angeles County Department of Health Services, 1999a). By October 1998, AIDS was third in reportable STDs; chlamydial infections and gonorrhea topped HIV infections among selected reportable diseases in Los Angeles County (Los Angeles County Department of Health Services, 1999b).

The dip in AIDS deaths is attributable to two factors. First, middle-aged homosexual/bisexual males are practicing safer sex. This group showed the greatest reduction (Fleming et al., 1998). Even IDUs showed declines in AIDS, though not as much in other groups ("Don't Let Up in War on AIDS," 1998). A factor linked to lower HIV/AIDS death rates is improved HIV/AIDS intervention/prevention programs, including education.

Second, declines in AIDS incidence and deaths in the United States are associated with the impact of treatment-induced delays in progression from HIV to AIDS and increased survival after diagnosis. New AIDS drugs have come into the market in recent years (Cimons, 1998). With treatments such as reverse transciptase inhibitors, which block an enzyme that enables the HIV to reproduce its genetic material, and protease inhibitors, which block another enzyme crucial for viral replication, some AIDS victims are living longer.

However, these drugs are expensive and many people do not have access to them. Their costs run about $1,200 per month. Furthermore, serious, annoying side effects have been reported which prevent some from taking the drugs (Read, 1999). The most effective treatment regimens have involved highly active anti-retroviral therapy, commonly known as HAART, which was introduced in 1995 (Williams et al., 1998). These are potent, so-called "triple cocktails" of two reverse transcriptase inhibitors and one protease inhibitor. Administration of such drugs has led to the observed decline in the annual and cumulative AIDS case fatality rate nationwide. However, after treatment with these drugs, which kill HIV, there are dormant viruses in cells that come back after the treatment has seemingly wiped out infection. An unintended consequence of these drugs has been a widely advertised public relations campaign with posters claiming that you can climb mountains with AIDS. People may feel that AIDS is not so bad—until they get infected.

Although these AIDS treatment drugs carry adverse side effects, with such treatments, hospitalizations and deaths of persons with AIDS have been reduced. Nonetheless, AIDS remains the leading cause of death for Americans twenty-five to forty-four years old and claims one life every eight minutes. A vaccine for AIDS prevention is not even close to being realized, according to most researchers. Tim Schacker, MD, is codirector of the clinical facility for AIDS patients and an assistant professor in the Department of Medicine at the University of Minnesota Medical School. This is one of twelve centers for AIDS research designated by the National Institutes of Health. Regarding an AIDS vaccine, Schacker says it "is not even on the horizon. There is some fundamental work that has to be done before we'll ever have a vaccine that will be useful for the world" (Read, 1999, p. 13).

The latest research involves "entry inhibition" drugs that block the very entrance of the HIV virus into cells. In contrast to reverse transcriptase inhibitors and protease inhibitors which block the action of two enzymes that HIV uses to take over cellular metabolism once the virus has invaded its target cells, entry inhibitors prevent the virus from entering the cell in the first place.

The "twilight of AIDS" has attracted wide attention, but the epidemic is not over (Rotello, 1996). Over the past couple of years, many people have become blasé and complacent, and think that AIDS is solved, that it is over, that the treatments are working, and that risk behavior in susceptible populations such as gays and IDUs is under control. But it is far from a done deal. There has only been a sort of temporary stay of execution.

## HEPATITIS C (HCV), A POTENTIALLY MORE SERIOUS HEALTH THREAT

In addition to AIDS, about 4 million Americans are infected with HCV in what health officials regard as a hidden epidemic (Centers for Disease Control and Prevention, 2001; Alter, 1997; Cimons, 1999). Hepatitis C, a blood-borne disease, is spread mostly by sexual contact and by IDU. In Riverside County, California, 24 percent of all jail inmates test positive for HCV. Preliminary reports show that about a third of all prisoners entering the California state prison system are infected ("HepC, Thriving on Ignorance," 2000). In Los Angeles County, in the two-month period of October-November 1999, compared with the same period in 1998, there was a threefold increase in reported cases of HCV (Los Angeles County Department of Health Services, 2000). Each year, about 180,000 Americans catch HCV. By way of comparison, 4 million Americans are HIV positive. Mickey Mantle died of HCV complications, and Evel Knievel has it. Many with HCV infection are asymptomatic, and the disease can smolder in the body for years without serious complications. Seventy percent of those infected do not realize that they have the disease because symptoms often do not appear for years, long after liver damage begins. Symptoms can be almost nonexistent and can include fatigue, loss of energy, and a slight loss of interest in life. The symptoms of hepatitis C are often very mild, at least in the early stages of infection, and can be virtually undetectable. It usually does not make itself known until the second or third decade of infection, often commencing with fatigue. When the disease process damages the liver badly enough, the symptoms become commensurate with cirrhosis and liver failure, including jaundice, abdominal swelling (ascites), and, finally, coma.

In Egypt, 15 percent of the entire population is now infected with HCV, and 100 million worldwide carry the virus. The sad news is that few of them will recover. HCV can cause chronic liver disease, cancer, and death. Hepatitis C—not alcoholism—is now the most common cause of cirrhosis of the liver. Still, HCV is not necessarily a death sentence—since only 20 percent of the people who are exposed to the virus go on to develop the most severe complications, and these may not occur until twenty or more years after initial infection.

Three out of four Americans have never heard of hepatitis C. Nor do most understand what kind of behavior puts them at greatest risk of exposure to HCV. HCV is different from the other two major hepatitis viruses. With hepatitis A, often spread through tainted food or unsanitary conditions, most individuals become ill but recover with the infection cleared from their bodies. With hepatitis B, most become ill but can recover, although 10 percent develop a persistent, chronic infection. This infection kills about 10,000 Americans annually.

Hepatitis C is far more contagious than HIV. Almost any direct or indirect exposure to infected blood can transmit HCV, such as giving someone with an open wound first aid, sharing a razor that nicked another person's face, or sharing works for injecting drugs.

Unquestionably, the most common cause of hepatitis C, accounting for about 50 percent of cases, is IDU. Intravenous drug users have prevalence rates of antibody to HCV (anti-HCV) exceeding 90 percent, higher than for any other group studied (Alter, 1995). HCV can be spread by sharing straws used for sniffing cocaine, a practice that can cause nasal bleeding. HCV also may be transmitted by sexual exposure to an infected person and exposure to multiple partners.

With HCV, as with HIV, gay men and promiscuous heterosexuals of either sex are significantly more vulnerable to infection. Persons like FSWs, with multiple sex partners, are at serious risk for HCV transmission and should follow safer sex practices, including using barriers (e.g., latex condoms) to prevent contact with body fluids. Low socioeconomic level is also a high-risk attribute of HCV.

Today there are effective vaccines available for hepatitis A and B, but none for HCV. Treatment for those with chronic hepatitis C is in its infancy. Only interferon, which helps only 15 to 20 percent of patients, has been used as a treatment. Interferon has all sorts of side effects: extreme pain, weight loss, lowered resistance to other diseases, overwhelming exhaustion, hair loss, low white blood cell count (leukopenia), and thyroid problems. Other, newer antiviral drugs are being tried in small clinical trials, along with nonpharmaceutical approaches. Most are aimed at reducing the amount of hepatitis C virus in the blood.

## REPORTED AIDS CASES IN MEXICO

Are Mexican street prostitutes at a higher risk for HIV exposure? The incidence and prevalence of HIV infection in Mexico is far lower than in the United States. As of December 1996, the Republic of Mexico—a nation of over 95 million—reported a total of 29,962 AIDS cases through their Sentinel Surveillance Registry of the National AIDS Council (Dirección Generál de Epidemiologia/CONASIDA, 1996; Rodríguez et al., 1998a).

Mexican incidence and prevalence surveys were performed between 1990-1997 in sixteen large- and medium-sized cities. A total sample of 17,105 men and 31,783 women were studied. They were recruited in HIV detection centers, on the streets, in STD clinics, public baths, and bars (Rodríguez et al. 1998a). By the end of 1997, 33,632 AIDS cases were registered in Mexico (Martinez, Magiz-Rodríguez, and Uribe-Zunga, 1998). AIDS/HIV infection in Mexico may be severely underreported (Ontiveros, personal communication; Velásquez, E., personal communication). The reported numbers suggest that the HIV/AIDS problem in Mexico is nowhere near the severity of the United States, or in some South Asian (Geeta, Lindan, and Hudes, 1995) and African (Kreiss et al., 1986; Piot et al., 1988) nations.

What are the major HIV/AIDS risk factors in Mexico and what is the HIV/AIDS rate? IDU accounts for a very much smaller proportion of HIV infection in Mexico than in the United States. According to the Mexican National Registry of AIDS Cases, 66 percent of all male cases are among homosexuals/bisexuals; only 1.1 percent of cases are attributed to IDU (Dirección General de Epidemiologia/CONASIDA, 1996; Velásquez, E., personal communication).

Among adult Mexican females, 50.2 percent of all AIDS cases develop from sex with infected males; 47 percent from transfusions with infected blood. A negligible .07 percent of female AIDS cases—less than one in a thousand—are attributed to IDU. In another study of 28,973 female sex workers conducted in eighteen Mexican states, the HIV seroprevalence rate was only 0.4 percent (Sandovál et al., 1998), extremely low compared with the United States. Typical HIV-positive rates of females enrolled in methadone maintenance clinics in Los Angeles run 6 to 7 percent. Even in a study of 350 IDUs in a Mexican prison in Tijuana, where 92 percent reported sharing needles/syringes, only 1.35 percent were HIV positive (Badillo et al., 1998).

Why, compared with American FSWs, are so few female AIDS cases in Mexico attributable to IDU, with prostitution as a secondary factor? A study of IDU rates and other HIV/AIDS risk behavior among Mexican street-level FSWs might provide some answers.

## THE RELATIONSHIP BETWEEN COMMERCIAL SEX WORK, AIDS, AND IDU

Although prostitution itself is a secondary risk factor for HIV infection in women (Piot et al., 1988; Von Reyn and Mann, 1987),

FSWs who are *IDUs* spread HIV and are *main transmitters* of the disease (Hagan and Gormley, 1998; Dicks, 1994). Among females, drug injection is the greatest risk factor for HIV infection (Booth, Crowley, and Zhang, 1996). IDU female street sex workers are exposed to a "double whammy" from HIV: infection by injecting drugs with contaminated hypodermic syringes and needles ("outfit," "works," "rig," etc.), and by multiple unprotected sexual contacts with seropositive clients and other IDUs.

Studies have shown significant differences in HIV seroprevalence between prostitutes who are IDUs or who engage in prostitution with IDUs and those who are not so exposed (Deren et al., 1997). Several reported investigations of African and European prostitutes demonstrate that those who share needles and other skin-penetrating instruments have high seropositivity rates (Clumeck et al., 1985; Denis et al., 1987; Kreiss et al., 1986; Nzilambi et al., 1988; Papaevengelou et al., 1985; Quinn et al., 1986; Sabatier, 1987; Tirelli et al., 1985; Van De Perre et al., 1985).

Variables related to HIV risk behaviors among prostitutes, such as IDU and unprotected sex, have included, (a) the professionalization of prostitution (brothel prostitutes display far lower rates of HIV infection than do street prostitutes); (b) the general geographic location of the industry (Eastern United States, Western Europe, South Asia, Central Africa, for example); and (c) specific locations where recruitment and prostitution activities occur (e.g., suburban/rural areas where seroprevalence is low, versus inner-city areas where infection rates are higher) (Deren et al., 1997).

Recent national studies of HIV seroprevalence reveal that most HIV-positive women in the United States are IDUs (CDC, 1995; Novick et al., 1989; Wofsy, 1988). The progressive chain of HIV infection among FSWs is generally (1) injected drug use; (2) prostitution for drug money; (3) HIV seropositivity. American female street sex workers may tend to use intravenous drugs, mainly heroin, because of certain personal traumas and factors in their lives. The stress involved in street work itself can contribute to IDU (Winick and Kinsie, 1971; Benjamin and Masters, 1964; Lewis, 1985; Millett, 1971).

Heroin-addicted female street sex workers are loose cannons in HIV transmission. The percentage of female IDU street sex workers who are HIV positive has ranged from about 4 percent in Los Angeles and San Diego (Ginsberg, personal interview, 1996; Bellis, 1993), to 80 percent in the mid-1980s in some major East Coast cities (Curran et al., 1988; CDC, 1985, 1986). In 1996, the seropositivity rate among street FSWs in Chicago was estimated at 35 percent (Buccholtz, personal interview, 1996). The overall HIV incidence rate among street-walking prostitutes in New York City during the period 1989-1995 was 31.3 percent (Wallace et al., 1996).

In 1997, 18 percent of female New York state prison entrants were HIV positive; most had IDU and commercial sex work histories. In FSWs (and with AIDS in women, generally) IDU is a more powerful predictor of HIV serostatus than multiple sex partners (Booth 1988a; Curran et al., 1988; CDC, 1987a; Kreiss et al., 1986). In San Bernardino, for example, most new AIDS cases among females (55 percent) result from IDU and heterosexual sex with an IDU partner (San Bernardino County, 2001). California is a major player in the distribution of drugs, heroin use is soaring to record high levels in the state, and San Bernardino is a transportation hub for illicit substances, including heroin and methamphetamine (San Bernardino Countywide Gangs and Drugs Task Force, 1998). Of California's fifty-eight counties, San Bernardino County ranks second in the rate of increasing heroin use (Maugh, 1998).

Chapter 3

# A Short History of Heroin
# and Commercial Sex Work

## *HEROIN*

All seventy-two Southern California FSWs interviewed for this book were heroin addicts. Is addiction associated with street prostitution? Does addiction cause prostitution, or does prostitution cause heroin addiction? What comes first, the hen or the egg? The drug/prostitution connection is one that continues to resist coherent analysis because cause and effect are difficult to distinguish. One analyst put it this way: "Prostitution provides support for drugs and drugs make it easier to prostitute" (James, 1976, p. 15). An addict-prostitute said:

> You can say prostitution feeds a drug habit. What comes first? Perhaps it's a kind of circle. You need the shit to kill the pain of prostitution; you need the prostitution to kill the pain of needing the drug. (Millett, 1971, p. 115)

For the FSW addicted to opiates, addiction necessitates continuing commercial sex work as the only possible means of supporting the habit which grows increasingly more expensive (my San Bernardino subjects used up to $350 worth a day) due to narcotic *tolerance.*

Heroin is derived from morphine base, which comes from opium. Opium is in the milky exudate obtained by incising the unripe seed pod of the poppy *(Papaver somniferum).* In 1805, a German pharmacist, Friedrich Sertürner, isolated an opium alkaloid he called morphine after the Greek god, Morpheus (god of dreams, son of Hypnos, the god of sleep).

The first hypodermic injections of morphine were given in America in 1856. Use of injected morphine increased during the Civil War to relieve pain from battlefield injuries; morphine addiction acquired the name "Soldiers Disease." By 1870 pharmaceutical manufacturing firms included huge doses of morphine in numerous proprietary medicines sold over the counter without prescription as household remedies. Sears Roebuck and Company advertised narcotic-injecting paraphernalia. No state or federal laws regulated sales and distribution of medicinal narcotic drugs. The addiction "problem" was regarded as more physiological than criminal. Typical addicts were middle-aged, white females who took narcotics to relieve menstrual cramps, diarrhea, or cough.

In 1874 the English chemist C.R. Wright first developed a semi-synthetic derivative of morphine, diacetylmorphine. In 1897, Heinrich Dreser, Head of the Pharmacological Institute of the Farbenfabriken vorm. Friedr. Bayer and Co. began pharmaceutical testing of the substance. He immediately coined the term "heroin" for the new drug because it performed so heroically in controlling pain—weight for weight it was three times more potent than morphine (Figure 3.1). By 1900, heroin was on the scene to stay, at first sold over the counter, then made illegal by the 1906 Pure Food and Drug Act and 1914 Harrison Narcotic Act.

The withdrawal syndrome in heroin addicts produces a combination of symptoms that are opposites of the acute effects. They include: nausea, diarrhea, coughing, yawning, lacrimation, rhinorrhea (runny nose), sweating, piloerection (goose bumps, the origin of the term quitting "cold turkey"), leg muscle contractions ("kicking the habit"), dysphoria, and intense drug craving. No deaths or serious complications from withdrawal have been reported in otherwise healthy persons (American Health Consultants, 2001).

David Musto, an eminent historian of narcotics control, suggested that the most passionate support for criminalization of narcotics was associated with fear of heroin's effect on specific minority groups in American society (Musto, 1973). It was especially feared because it seemed to undermine social restrictions which were essential to keep these groups—mainly African Americans, Mexican and Asian immigrants—under control. The Harrison Narcotic Act laid the legal foundation for the punitive approach to the narcotics problem, including its black market economics (Musto, 1973; Duster, 1970; Bellis, 1983) as addicts were forced to underground sources for their drug supplies.

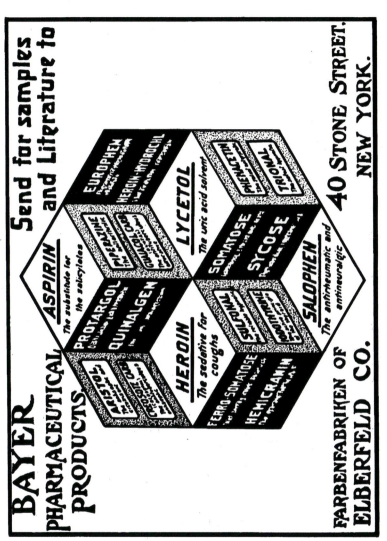

FIGURE 3.1. Bayer heroin advertisement, circa 1900. Available over the counter, no prescription required. (Used by permission of Bayer AG. West Germany)

In a blaze of enlightenment, narcotic *maintenance* clinics (a portent of today's methadone maintenance programs) were briefly opened between 1919 and 1923. Reports at the time noted their success in reducing crimes to obtain drugs (U.S. Commissioner of Internal Revenue, 1921; New York City Health Department, 1920).

Amidst media-inspired public indignation and government propaganda against the narcotic maintenance clinics ("No to Re-Opening Narcotics Clinic," 1938; "State Should Not Take Over Selling Dope," 1938), all forty-four clinics in America were closed by the mid-1920s. The fear that the enemies of the United States were trying to flood the nation with drugs in order to sap our "moral fiber" or destroy our youth is one that "drug czar" Harry Anslinger played on during WWII, and one that has underlain U.S. drug policy ever since. Anslinger, later to direct the first Federal Bureau of Narcotics (then becoming chief of the Bureau of Narcotics and Dangerous Drugs, now in its most recent incarnation, the Drug Enforcement Administration), was a vocal proponent of the clinic closures (Anslinger and Tomkins, 1953). Again, addicts turned to crimes such as prostitution for money to obtain their now illicit—and very expensive—narcotics. Thus, the situation has remained until this day.

The term addiction is not easily defined, but in all cases it manifests itself in the twin phenomena of *tolerance* and *physical dependence*. Tolerance refers to the situation wherein after repeated administration of a drug, higher doses are required to elicit effects previously produced by smaller doses. Physical dependence is characterized by withdrawal symptoms when chronic use of an addictive drug is discontinued: For the severe opiate addict there is the juggernaut of extreme anxiety, insomnia, craving for narcotics, sweating, increased respiratory rate, fever, chills, goose flesh, dilated pupils, cramping, explosive diarrhea and vomiting, almost unbearable pains, and the relentless craving or "yen" for more heroin to relieve these symptoms (Hodding, Jann, and Ackerman, 1980). Only another solid dose of narcotics, preferably administered intravenously, gives relief. Given this "Algebra of Need," as William Burroughs (1959) phrased it, heroin is quantitative and easily measurable: the more you have the more you use, and the more you use, the less you have. Its use jousts with need. Heroin is thus the ideal consumer product, the ultimate merchandise. No sales talk is necessary between user and connection: the addict will crawl through a sewer and beg to buy. This is why, in economic terms, demand for heroin is relatively price inelastic: addicts have a physical or powerful psychological need for the drug and their level of use tends to be driven by their needs rather than the price.

Prostitution, particularly in its street variety, is intimately associated with drug abuse. Injected drug use, mainly heroin, is common among such women.

## DEFINITIONS OF PROSTITUTION

There are as many definitions of the prostitute and prostitution as there are writers on the subject, but they basically boil down to,

> any sexual acts, including those which do not actively involve copulation, habitually performed by individuals with other individuals of their own or the opposite sex, for a consideration which is non-sexual. (Henriques, 1963, p. 17)

The elements that seem common to prostitution are promiscuousness, pecuniary reward, professional commercialism, and a special type of person (Bullough, 1964). Other commonalities include absence of emotional involvement between provider and client, frequent sexual contacts, exclusively sexual outlets, a temporary relationship, and cash as the usual consideration for services (Decker, 1979).

Female commercial sex work is the granting of commercial sexual access, established by mutual consent of the woman, her client, and/or her employer, for remuneration which provides part or all of her livelihood. In California, the state penal code (PC647(a)) defines it as, "Any lewd act between persons for money or other consideration." The state of Washington says that a "person is guilty of prostitution if that person engages or agrees or offers to engage in sexual conduct with a person in return for a fee" (RCW 9A.88.030). A simpler definition is the giving or receiving of the body for sex acts for hire (Winick and Kinsie, 1971). The exchange of money between the customer and commercial sex worker, in most cases, legally distinguishes the commercial sex server from the merely promiscuous male or female.

Sexual intercourse with commercial sex workers, as distinguished from sex under almost any other conditions, is unique by virtue of the fact that each coition or extracoital act is paid for separately and at the time, and usually in cash. Another characteristic of the typical sex worker-customer relationship, compared to most other sexual relationships, is its transience (and, usually, brevity). Relations are generally temporary (Decker, 1979). Ordinarily, only the customer is motivated by a desire for sexual pleasure.

Various terms have been used to label commercial sex workers, including harlot, hooker (after the "camp followers" of General Joseph Hooker during the Civil War), prostitute, whore, stroller, and streetwalker. Types of FSWs have been categorized: call girls, streetwalkers, bar prostitutes, brothel prostitutes, dance hall and exotic dancer or stripper prostitutes, massage parlor sex workers, escort service prostitutes, homeless prostitutes, elderly prostitutes, transsexual and transvestite prostitutes, homosexual prostitutes, and child prostitutes.

Recently, more neutral, industrially oriented labels have been employed: commercial sex workers, female sex workers, and sex servers. "Sex worker" is the term preferred by many in the industry to the old-fashioned "prostitute" or derogatory "hooker." The prostitution business now is known as part of a wider "sex industry," which also includes pornographic tapes and films, sex aids, the online adult industry, nude dance clubs, pornographic film/video parlors, massage parlors, and escort services, among other outlets. Major Mexican daily newspapers today refer more neutrally to *sexoservidores* (sex servers), not *prostitutas*.

"Streetwalking" (L: *ambulatrices,* strollers) is probably the most ancient of FSW operating methods. This approach is also most objectionable to many persons, because of the streetwalker's high degree of visibility. Historically, since earliest times, the streetwalker has been regarded as being at or near the bottom of the sex work ladder. Her fees have traditionally been lower than those received by most other types of sex servers, and she has been, in general, a less attractive type, usually attributable to the rigors of her mode of operation and drug misuse. Also, in general, the venereal disease rate is higher among streetwalkers than among "call girls," sex workers in brothels such as those in Nevada, and bar prostitutes. The streetwalker is most likely to be victimized by dangerous sexual deviates. Regularly, such women are the targets of rapes, beatings, and serial killers. They also are the most exposed to the police; known prostitutes are much more easily harassed and arrested when streetwalking.

Occupying the lowest rung of this commercial sex ladder in both Mexico and the United States is the street trade. These types of women have hit bottom. They represent about 10 to 20 percent of all FSWs. Lower-class street FSWs have the worst working conditions of any sex workers, earn the least money, and must cope with contempt all the way up the judgmental ladder, from residents and business-people around their working areas, from the criminal justice system, and from their relatives (Alexander, Highleyman, and La Croix, 1996; City and County of San Francisco, 1996; Symanski, 1981). Police discriminate against street FSWs more than any other types of prostitutes because they are the most visible (City and County of San Francisco, 1996).

Street sex workers were interviewed for this book because the street trade is at the bottom of the scale in the prostitution hierarchy (Lewis, 1985). Predictors of prostitution are found in various domains, from family, community, and peers, to individual factors such as negative life events and early childhood sexual abuse. Street-walkers are subjected to the most stress, and seem statistically most likely to be IDUs and at risk for HIV transmission.

Interest in what these women at the bottom of the sex trade knew about AIDS, and if fear of the disease caused them to alter their drug use and sexual behavior sparked the writing of this book.

## HISTORY OF PROSTITUTION

Commercial sex work flourished in ancient Rome, Cyprus, Babylon, Egypt, among the Canaanites, and in ancient Greece. Philosophers such as Socrates, Plato, Diogenes, and Praxiteles enjoyed the company of prostitutes, the highest class of whom were known as *hetaerae,* the prostitute class. A large number of *hetaerae* who were thought of as sacred worked at Aphrodite's sanctuary on the Acro-cornith in Athens. They held splendid ceremonies in honor of Aphrodite and often posed half or fully naked as models for statues of Aphrodite (Mavromataki, 1997). In the middle, below the elite *hetaerae,* were the *auletrides,* or flute players. Ancient streetwalkers of Athens occupied the lowest rung of the ladder. Generally, prostitution was given high status in ancient Greece. Historical data demonstrate the overwhelming significance of commercial sex work in large places—cities, for which Greece's city states were famous.

The Roman approach to commercial sex work was somewhat like our own: periods of toleration countered by epochs of (unsuccessful) prohibition. Hypocritical Roman politicians rose from the embraces of sex workers to rail against vice and the decline of public morality, reminiscent of some of today's legislators who vote to criminalize commercial sex work while utilizing the services of the criminal class they created.

The first known regulation of prostitution in Europe dates from Rome. A woman wishing to follow the profession appeared before an official. She had to give her name, age, and birthplace. These data were inscribed on a roll, and she was given a license, *licentia stupre*. She also had to state how much she would charge, which was also noted on the roll (Henriques, 1963). Patrician women were absolutely forbidden to act as prostitutes. Brothels were open to inspection by officials at all times. Disorderly behavior was terminated by arrest and punishment. Brothelkeepers who failed to register workers could be fined. Prostitutes were offered protection against clients who tried to bilk them of their proper fees. All was conducted with "proper decorum" (Henriques, 1963). There were two categories of Roman prostitutes: registered (those who paid the tax) and unregistered. In Rome, numerous divisions and subdivisions existed among *prostibulae: Delicatae* and *Famosae* at the top. They were the equivalent of the Greek *hetaerae*. Streetwalkers were known as *ambulatrices notilucae*. At the very bottom of the Roman sex work mountain were *quadrantariae,* who could be had for less than a penny.

The prostitute was an established part of ancient Indian life 5,000 years ago, in ancient China, and the Arab world. In India, control was exercised through a system of regulation similar to the European version.

Prostitution was omnipresent during the Middle Ages when the leading fathers of the Christian church tolerated and even sanctioned prostitution (Henriques, 1963). Pope Alexander VI repeatedly entertained prostitutes in the Vatican palace, and other Popes taxed prostitutes. King Louis IX, the religious king of France, tried to suppress prostitution, but his edicts were about as effective as the Volstead (1919, repealed in 1933) and Harrison Narcotic (1914) Acts in the

United States. Martin Luther was outspoken against prostitution, but today, prostitution is legal in Germany and carefully controlled.

In Western society, widespread antiprostitution sentiment began to arise in the 1500s. By the sixteenth century, when an epidemic of syphilis swept Europe, the brothels were blamed and closed. Sexually transmitted diseases were widespread in the Middle Ages, and although their causes were unknown, it was believed that the brothels contributed to their incidence and prevalence. During the Italian Renaissance, sex work flourished, especially in cities: Rome, Naples, Venice, Florence, and Bologna. In 1490 there were an estimated 6,800 registered prostitutes and many other clandestine ones in Rome (out of a total city population of 90,000). It was not until the sixteenth century, when venereal diseases began to claim a fearsome toll in Italy and elsewhere, that an authentic antipathy toward prostitution became widespread and gained influence.

Prostitution existed among early Native Americans who serviced European colonists. When Africans were brought as slaves to America, they gradually and largely replaced Native Americans in that capacity. Benjamin Franklin and Thomas Jefferson purchased African slaves and used them for sexual pleasure (these were more "sex slaves" than prostitutes). The last half of the nineteenth century and early part of the twentieth century may be regarded as the "golden age" of the brothel in America. Pimps arranged for the rental of rooms, paid fines, bribed local politicos and police, took care of unruly customers, brought in trade, and otherwise made themselves useful.

## THE FSW HIERARCHY AND THE BOTTOM RUNG OF THE LADDER

Almost everyone knows the status hierarchy in commercial sex work: At the pinnacle are expensive "call girls." They tend to see themselves at the "top of the profession" (Ignoto, 1999). Their self-concept is that they are the best looking, best trained, and most selective sex workers. At hotels in Las Vegas, some earn $5,000 a night servicing wealthy businessmen, or "high rollers," who, at that price, do not tolerate alcohol and drug use.

Escort services rate just below call girls. The Manhattan yellow pages list about twenty pages of massage and escort outfits, serving mostly businesspeople and tourists. Los Angeles has the "Creme De La Creme" (sic) and "Freelance Models" escort services. These escorts specialize in almost everything, from "massage, nude modeling, and fantasies," to "lingerie and topless." Today, the Mexico City phone directory contains five pages of these listings. High-dollar escorts, if arrested on prostitution charges, tend to have lawyers who obtain reduced sentences. No such option exists for street workers.

Beverly Hills ex-madam Elizabeth "Alex" Adams, Los Angeles's Heidi Fleiss, and Jody Diane "Babydol" Gibson are madams who have hired out aspiring actresses and other high-end "escorts." Gibson advertised on the Web. Fleiss, who served time for tax evasion and pandering, and a one-time Gibson competitor, said that Babydol Gibson's sex workers were older, with a less prestigious address and clientele. Whereas Gibson's women charged $500 to $3,000 for a date, Fleiss's rock-bottom price was $1,500, and most of her clients paid three or four times that, depending on the length of the date. The common price for perfectly legal street sex in Mexico was about $4 (in 2001). The Los Angeles Police Department goes after prostitution cases when they meet the three Cs: "commercial, conspicuous, and complained about" (Lait and Hubler, 1999). Babydol Gibson got a three-year prison term in May, 2000 for operating her high-priced international prostitution ring that catered to celebrities, politicians, and wealthy businessmen (Haynes, 2000).

Next on the ladder are legal "brothel sex workers," who can be found only in the United States in ten out of seventeen Nevada counties where commercial sex is legal. Since 1971, Nevada counties of fewer than 400,000 population have had the option of electing to legalize brothels such as the Mustang Ranch near Reno, Nevada. At present, a total of thirty-two Nevada brothels employ about 300 licensed prostitutes. They go by names such as the Moonlite Bunnyranch, the Cherry Patch, and the Chicken Ranch in Pahrump, Nevada. In 1998, local Nevada governments collected over $500,000 from brothel licenses and associated fees (Platt, 2001).

The typical employment situation in Nevada's brothels is a contractual arrangement between the women and the owners (not unlike much employment now in the United States). In this way, brothel owners avoid paying employee-related taxes and giving their "girls" health insurance, sick leave, and workers' compensation. Typically, managers prohibit the women from leaving the grounds while on

duty, and often listen to their private negotiations with clients over secret intercom systems to discourage the women from withholding
part of management's cut or trade sex for drugs.

Brothel sex workers in these operations undergo weekly, state-
mandated medical examinations for gonorrhea, herpes, condyloma
lata (venereal warts, due to syphilis) and monthly blood tests for
syphilis. AIDS testing began in 1986. They are tested for HIV each
month. Between July 1, 1988, and December 31, 1993, more than
20,000 HIV tests were conducted among these workers. *None* of the
women employed at *any* of the Nevada brothels were HIV positive
(Platt, 2001). In another recent study of forty-four Nevada brothel sex
workers (Albert et al. 1995), *all* women reported using a condom for
*every* act of vaginal intercourse with a brothel client in the previous
year. The absence of HIV and other STDs among these women may
be explained by the fact that clients are required under Nevada state
law to use condoms during every sex act.

A notch down from the Vegas-type call girls, escorts, and legal
brothel prostitutes in Nevada are the "bar sex workers" and those who
transact business within massage parlors, and "outcall massage workers." A listing in the San Francisco yellow pages reads "San Francisco Outcall Massage."

Bar prostitutes are common in Mexican red-light districts. Americans who go to Mexico for prostitutes call these zones "boys town."
Some of the bars are discos, others have strippers, but most are simply Mexican honky-tonk bars where the sex servers wait for customers to buy them a drink, dance, and lock down the sex deal.

In the United States, some club strippers and exotic dancers also
practice commercial sex work. Their fees are in the $100-500 range,
and sex services are usually provided at a location other than the club.
Also popular today are strippers and nude dancers who provide private entertainment at the clients' location of choice. They are popular
for bachelor parties. At the Lusty Lady theater in San Francisco, recently the site of a bitter—and ultimately successful—unionization
campaign, Miss Mary Ann, a peep-show dancer complained,

> The job has always been defined in MY mind by the repetitive
> manual labor it demands. . . . Make eye contact, pout, wink,
> swivel your hips a little . . . fondle your tits, smack your ass,
> stroke whatever pubic hair you haven't shaven off, repeat these
> ten steps until the customer comes . . . (quoted in Platt, 2001, p. 6)

# Chapter 4

# Study Setting and Methods

## *WHY MEXICO?*

Mexico has 8,000 years of cultural development, with fifty-six distinct ancient ethnic groups including Zapotecos, Mixtecos, Huaves, Tarahumaras, Chocos, Nahuas, and Mayas. Mexico today, a nation of over 92 million people ("Crisis y Demografia," 1998) and thirty-three states, is a major drug-producing and exporting country, as are Peru, Bolivia, Colombia, Thailand, Laos, Myanmar, Afghanistan, Pakistan, Turkey, and Iran. According to the Mexican government itself, "the most perverse effect and the most important change that the drug market has introduced to Mexican society is the violence that drug trafficking breeds" (Toro, 1995, p. 57).

Mexico's drug problem is not so much illicit drug consumption as it is the social overhead costs imposed by two unfortunate conditions: prohibition in the United States, which drives prices up, and Mexico's border status with the world's largest illegal drug market. The real source of the drug problem in the United States lies within ourselves, and our own society. All vice control efforts are susceptible to corruption, but none so much as drug enforcement. What makes drug enforcement especially vulnerable to corruption are the astronomical amounts of money involved in the business.

Mexico still is not a country in which consumption of drugs is a major problem. In a 1988 Mexican national household drug use survey, it was found that the prevalence of use in Mexico was less than one-tenth that in the United States (Dirección Generál de Epidemiologia and Instituto Mexicano de Psiquiatria, 1989). This survey showed that the highest percentage of drug use in Mexico among adults is for marijuana. Of the entire Mexican population, regular heroin use was reported as "insignificant." The fact is, Mexicans are so poor that the price of heroin and cocaine cannot be met by the average Mexicano. Perceived availability has not correlated strongly with drug use in Mexico.

Nonetheless, Mexico is reputedly a *narcoestado*—a veritable drug-state ("Mexico no es Narcoestado," 1998). The drug cartels have penetrated the Mexican state and its socioeconomic structures so deeply that they have effectively subverted most of the country's major institutions. The upper and lower houses of the Mexican Congress and the executive branch, state governors, banks, businesses, the criminal justice system—have all, to one extent or another, been corrupted. The Federal Judicial Police is so corrupt that it is no longer possible to distinguish between them and the criminals they are supposed to apprehend. In fact, some of these police officials protect the drug rackets.*

Violence, and the collusion of Mexican officials in drug trafficking, goes back to 1910 (Walker, 1981), spurred largely by the U.S. Pure Food and Drug Act and the Harrison Narcotic Acts which prohibited heroin and marijuana in the United States. These prohibition policies drove up drug prices, thus making production and trafficking a lucrative business in Mexico.

By 1975, Mexico was supplying around 87 percent of the heroin and nearly 95 percent of the marijuana consumed in the United States (Toro, 1995). Stiffer antidrug law enforcement, particularly eradication and interdiction programs in Mexico pushed by U.S. officials, tend to have a "cartelization" effect on the market. Interdiction source control is largely unable to keep illicit drugs out of the United States. Interdiction policies and programs push less daring and smaller traffickers out of the business, consequently benefiting the most powerful and organized.

Mexico has a list of violent cartels—the Tijuana cartel, the Juárez cartel, the Gulf cartel, the Jalisco cartel, and more that foster the complicity of Mexican authorities. The cartels have moved into the Yucatán Peninsula, which was previously free of the grip of those cartels dominating the Mexican states that border the United States.

In Cancún, Quintana Roo, known for its upscale hotels, crystal beaches, and MTV youth parties, Italian mafia members have teamed

---

*Mexico's officialdom should not be singled out here. U.S. interventions in various countries, especially in Asian, Afghani, Turkish, Nicaraguan, and Mexican politics, have played major roles in shaping trends in the world heroin and cocaine industries (Webb, 1998; Cockburn and St. Clair, 1998; Levine, 1998; Reinarman and Levine, 1998; McCoy, 1972).

up with lieutenants of the dead Juárez cartel boss, Amado Carrillo Flores, to smuggle cocaine and launder drug money. The ex-governor of Quintana Roo, Mário Villanueva, accused of protecting the traffickers, denied any links with the drug trade calling such allegations "politically motivated slander" (Sheridan, 1998c, p. A1). In April 1999, the day after ending his six-year term, and in an embarrassing blow to Mexico's justice system, Villanueva went into hiding to avoid being jailed (Sheridan, 1999). The U.S. Drug Enforcement Administration said he was a key figure in turning the Yucatán Peninsula into a major entryway for U.S.-bound cocaine. He finally was nabbed in 2001 under the administration of Vicente Fox.

Crop eradication is the backbone of Mexican drug control policy, but organized traffickers have always found ways to cultivate drugs such as opium poppies and marijuana. "Mary Jane" is the Americanized word for "*Juana* Jane," or, marijuana.

The Mexican drug trade is estimated, at minimum, to be a $40 billion dollar-a-year business. Mexican oil sales (the nation's biggest legal export) pale by comparison, bringing in only $7 billion (Macella and Schulz, 1997).

Mexican government officials at all levels are routinely tied to the illicit drug trade, though they regularly deny such connections. According to Mexican Special Prosecutor for Attention to Crimes Against Public Health Mariano Herran Salvatti, "There is not one person in the executive branch of this country who is connected in any way to narcotic trafficking" ("Mexico no es Narcoestada," 1998, p. A26). Average Mexicans laugh at this, but Mexican officials such as Herran Salvatti maintain that the United States must share blame for the drug problem: as Mexico cannot control the production of illegal drugs, the United States cannot control its consumption.

In 1987, drug trafficking was declared a national security problem for the first time by former Mexican President Miguel de la Madríd. Former President Carlos Salinas de Gortarí defined the problem in the same terms, but his brother, Raul Salinas de Gortarí, has been accused of *lavado de dinero*—drug money laundering, and of literally opening up the gates of the drug flow from Mexico into the United States (Dahlberg and Sheridan, 1998; De Córdoba and Studer, 1998).

In a 369-page report by authorities in Switzerland, where Raul Salinas kept secret accounts, it was alleged that, after his younger brother was elected president, Raul Salinas de Gortarí took personal control of practically all drug shipments transiting Mexico. By demanding cuts of up to 40 percent of the drugs' value, he pocketed at least $500 million in illicit drug profits, which were paid to guarantee the security of tons of cocaine passing through Mexico. He provided trucks and even railroad freight cars from state-owned enterprises to speed the illegal cocaine cargoes. Bribes were paid to cooperating members of the Mexican police and army (Dahlberg and Sheridan, 1998). Predictably, Salinas' attorney said that these reports about his client were "absolutely false" ("Salinas Kin Linked to Cocaine," 1998).

Raul Salinas met his fate in 1999 when he was convicted of the assassination of his brother-in-law, Francisco Ruiz Massieu, the number-two man in Mexico's ruling PRI (Partido Revolucionario Institucional) party and former governor of the drug-producing state of Guerrero. Salinas was sentenced to fifty years in Mexican prison (Sheridan and Smith, 1999). He could die there, but could also win his case on appeal.

Mexico's president at this writing, Vicente Fox (ex-Coca-Cola executive), like his immediate predecessor Ernesto Zedillo Ponce de Leon (son of an army general), continues to identify narco-trafficking as the primary threat to Mexican national security.

Recently, in "Operation Casablanca," U.S. drug enforcement agents gathered criminal information on numerous large Mexican banks allegedly laundering money from drug profits through electronic transfers to their consorts in the United States ("Lavaron Once Bancos 55 Milliones de Dólares," 1998). The United States carried out part of this undercover sting operation on Mexico soil without Mexican authorization on the grounds that Mexicans could not be trusted with the information. Most of the drug money gathered by Mexican traffickers is spent and laundered in the United States (Maingot, 1988). Schemes to launder drug money include mixing illegal money with legal cash from supermarkets, restaurants, real estate, *casas de cambio* (money exchanges), or buying chips and cashing them in Las Vegas and other gambling centers.

Twenty-two big Mexican banks were under suspicion in the Operation Casablanca money-laundering racket. Operation Casablanca was a three-year investigation of money laundering activities of Colombia's Cali drug cartel and the Juárez cartel in Mexico. U.S. federal prosecutors reported that tens of millions of dollars were laundered through phony transactions to the Mexican-owned banks. The money was supplied to the banks through a government informant and undercover U.S. Customs Service agents operating out of a storefront in Santa Fe Springs, California. During the operation, the bankers were told, usually, as they visited Santa Fe Springs, that the money came from Colombia's Cali drug cartel. The sting operation also included a former member of Mexico's Juárez cartel who helped recruit the bankers.

Ultimately, the total number of convictions in the case came to forty, while more than sixty individuals remain fugitives (Krasnowski, 1999). In the end, three of the banks were finally indicted by the U.S. Justice Department and pleaded guilty to criminal charges in 1999: Bancomér and Banca Serfín, Mexico's second- and third-largest banks, respectively, and the smaller Confia bank. The banks paid over $15 million in fines (Rosenzweig, 1999a). Newspapers described the money laundering scheme, linked to the Juárez drug cartel, as the biggest drug money laundering case ever (Rosenzweig, 1999b).

The Mexican press pointedly accused "American police agents" in Mexico working on the Operation Casablanca case as representing a "violation of national sovereignty" ("Lavaron Once Bancos 55 Milliones de Dólares," 1998, p. 1-A). The Mexican government reacted angrily. Former Mexican President Zedillo urged, "We must all respect the sovereignty of each nation so that no one can become the judge of others and no one feels the need to violate other countries' laws for the sake of enforcing its own" (Bertram and Sharpe, 1998, p. M2).

Painting Mexico as an unreliable ally in the drug war threatens other U.S. interests. Good-neighbor relations with Mexico are essential to protect the commerce created by free trade and the steady flow of investments, loans, tourists, oil, and immigrant labor between the two countries. Former U.S. Attorney General Janet Reno was quick to smooth Mexican feathers over Operation Casablanca, stating apologetically,

> only three banks were incriminated in the money laundering scheme and I want to assure [Mexico] that this does not incriminate all banks in Mexico. I want to make this very clear. [The Mexican Attorney General and Treasury Secretary] are dedicated to ensuring that Mexican laws against money laundering

are implemented as they are in the United States. ("Exonera Publicamente EU al Sistema," 1998, p. 10-A)

Former Secretary of State Madeleine Albright also soothed Mexican officials by chastising Treasury Secretary Robert Rubin for failing to inform her about the money-laundering sting operation in Mexico. In a letter to Rubin Albright said that, "I would appreciate being kept personally informed of developing investigations in Mexico and other foreign countries that could have a significant foreign policy fallout" ("Mexico Sting Irks Secretary," 1998).

Police units in Mexico have been the most vulnerable to corruption: sooner or later they seem to develop links with traffickers. Police units in Mexico have had to be disbanded periodically because of their collusion with drug traffickers. New units are set up to replace or oversee existing ones. Such is the case with the recently created Federal Preventive Police. In an ostensible effort to fight drugs, corruption, and to regain public trust, this new unit brings together the federal highway police (widely regarded as the most honest police agency in Mexico), immigration officials, and customs agents into a single operation. Agents receive substantially higher wages than those of regular police (Gaza, 1999).

Mexico has 4,480 police agencies, compared with 18,769 in the United States (U.S. Department of Justice, 1998). In Mexico, 2,380 of the departments are municipal and thirty-three are state judicial and federal police units. There are also other police units—the "Metro" in Mexico City, the mounted police, the rural police, the federal military police, the naval, the auxiliary, and the bank police, the fiscal police, and more than 1,000 corporate providers of security services, all of whom are under suspicion of being "on the take." Mexico City, the most populated city on the planet, has 70,000 police officers (Pick and Butler, 1997).

Half of all Mexican civilian police have not completed grade school, and the average salary of a city police officer is $120 U.S. per month. In contrast, starting salaries for local police officers in the United States as of 1997 averaged about $2,300 a month, with officers in larger departments averaging $2,550 a month in starting pay (U.S. Department of Justice, 1999). A commander in the Mexico City police with twenty-plus years on the force brings home $960 U.S. a month; the comparable position in a small-city police department in the United States (such as Fontana, California) is *$6,500 a month.*

Such low salaries are a strong inducement for Mexican *policia* to involve themselves with the drug trade, especially bribery and extortion in return for protection.

According to the Forensic Medical Service in Mexico City, an average of 15.1 cadavers per day are brought in, of which 99 percent are referred to the prosecutor's office as suspicious deaths. A total of 3.3 violent homicides related to the drug trade occur per day in Mexico City—caused by gunshot, beatings, and strangulation ("No Coinciden con la Información," 1998). As in the United States, Mexico cannot get a handle on its own *guerra contra las drugas* (drug war). Although Mexican officials claim that they are on a "fast track" in combating narco traffickers, their *uniformados* are always implicated in various forms of corruption, much of it involving the illicit drug trade.

The drug war is also corrupting the Mexican army. U.S. officials pushed former President Zedillo to call in the army to replace the civilian police, widely seen as corrupt. Under the plan, the military would get tough with the drug traffickers, and its more professional image would play well in the United States. Former President Zedillo responded to U.S. pressure by calling in the military. In December 1996, generals were put in charge of the Mexican Federal Judicial Police, the National Institute to Combat Drugs, and the Center for Planning for Drug Control. Military personnel have also occupied top law enforcement posts in two-thirds of Mexico's states.

Former President Zedillo appointed Army General Jesús Gutierrez Rebollo as head of the Instituto Nacionál para el Combate a las Drugas, the Mexican counterpart of the U.S.'s General Barry McCaffrey, director of the White House Office of National Drug Control Policy. General Gutierrez Rebollo had been packaged as a step forward. His appointment was part of a much-trumpeted move by former President Zedillo to draft the military into antidrug enforcement after the ineffectiveness and corruption of the civilian police force became overwhelming. U.S. drug policy director McCaffrey hailed Gutierrez as a man of great "integrity . . . patriotic, honest, dedicated" (Bertram and Shapre, 1998, p. M2).

Gutierrez Rebollo was brought in to rebuild the previous antidrug agency—which had been created to replace *its* corrupt predecessor. However, in 1997, ten generals and twenty-two other military officers were under investigation for alleged ties to traffickers (Bertram and Sharpe, 1998). Ironically, Gutierrez Rebollo himself, Mexico's top antinarcotics official, was arrested in February 1997, convicted, and sentenced for selling protection to one of the country's most powerful drug lords.

After his arrest, a new organized crime unit was created with much fanfare. Again, the names of fifteen officers from the U.S.-trained Organized Crime Unit within the Mexican attorney general's office were found in documents seized from drug traffickers in mid-1998; five were fired when they failed lie-detector tests (Bertram and Sharpe, 1999).

Mexican critics of the drug war call all of this *corrupción institucionalizada*—institutionalized corruption. As a top Mexican newspaper opined: "Mexico is a country of generalized corruption, saturated by the narco traffickers. It involves the grave corrosion of the structures of the Mexican state. The fundamental national problem is organized crime" ("El Problema Fundamentál," 1998, p. 4).

The realities of the "war on drugs" have dragged the Mexican government into a spiral of increasingly punitive programs that have rendered the manufacture and smuggling of drugs more (rather than less) appealing and the organization of this illegal market a threat to civilized and effective governance. The current policy of over-criminalization is not working.

A lot of thought went into a research trip to Mexico to interview street sex workers in seamy parts of various cities. The perceived crime wave in Mexico, much of it related to drugs, has spawned what the U.S. State Department and Mexican officials refer to as *El problema de la inseguridád turística en México* (the tourist insecurity problem in Mexico). Except for the glitzy tourist meccas along the Pacific Riviera such as Acapulco, Puerto Vallarta, Mazatlán, and Gulf destinations such as Cozumél and Cancún, the American tourist trade dropped off significantly in the 1990s. Widely circulated reports of Americans killed by *machetazo* (hacked to death), kidnapped, and arrested in Mexico have led most Americans to think twice about venturing into the country's interior, especially in cars or R.V.'s. Mexico City's largest newspaper reports, "Newspaper reports on poor air quality, the wave of assaults, assassinations, as well as highway bandits and kidnappings, are inhibiting tourism [to Mexico] ("Exonera Pulicamente," 1998, p. 10A).

In 1998 the *Los Angeles Times* reported,

> Two Northern Nevada men, who hadn't been heard from since
> the second day of a planned two-week fishing trip to Mexico in
> November, have been found dead in Baja California. . . . The
> men [were] reported killed by sharp blows to the head. . . .
> (Thomas, 1998, p. C-8)

Reports such as these have struck fear in Americans' hearts and have
hurt tourism in Mexico.

The "crime wave" in Mexico never surfaced while conducting research for this book. It seems largely confined to Mexicans who live
in really tough urban neighborhoods such as the Iztapalapa and
Nezahualcoyótl districts in Mexico City. Nezahualcoyótl, the im-
mense, garbage-strewn, eastern bedroom suburb in the state of Mexico built on the dry bed of Lake Texcoco, just beyond the federal district's border, is named for an Aztec poet king of the 1400s. Its
population of 3 million consists largely of indigenous people who
have migrated to the metropolis from rural villages. Crime is also
largely representative of internecine warfare between *las organ-
izaciones criminales*—organized criminal gangs involved in drug
production and trafficking, and to visitors who flaunt large bills and
expensive watches, drive at night, or who are themselves involved in
heavy drinking or illicit drug activities.

American pressure on Mexico to step up drug interdiction affords
numerous face-to-face contacts with Mexican law enforcement officials. Enhanced law enforcement is apparent all over the country.
Crossing the border at Ciudad Juárez when entering Mexico used to
be a simple "wave through." Now there are detailed examinations of
Mexican and American vehicles which look for illegal firearms, cash,
drugs, even toilets or lumber that can be purchased more cheaply on
the American side of the border at Home Depot discount stores. Mexican "fiscal police" want Mexican nationals to "buy Mexican." On the
main highways, roadblocks manned by Mexican army troops, complete with battle fatigues and automatic weapons with banana clips
are prevalent. Mexican federal and state judicial police with drug-
sniffing dogs are also present at some roadblocks. Today, some 40
percent of the 180,000-member Mexican army is reportedly working
on drug control (Bertram and Sharpe, 1999). Mexico is about the
only Latin American country where leftist insurgents untainted (so

far) by the drug trade can be found facing down counterinsurgent forces equipped with U.S. drug-control dollars.

All of this indicates the pressure from the United States and upper echelons of Mexican officialdom to uncover illegal activities, especially drug transhipments. The nagging paradox is that the more efficient the Mexican police and military become because of U.S. pressure, training, and equipment, the better able they are to track and find traffickers, and the higher the bribes they can extract. In addition, the success in increasing the cost of trafficking has raised U.S. street drug prices, generating huge profits for producers and traffickers.

## *WHY PARTICULAR MEXICAN CITIES WERE CHOSEN IN WHICH TO INTERVIEW PROSTITUTES*

Why Tijuana for street prostitute interviews? First, the state of Baja California Norte has the second highest reported rate (cases per million) of AIDS cases in Mexico (after Mexico City) (Ellingwood, 2000a). In addition, the incidence of AIDS in the San Diego and Tijuana region is the highest of any stretch of the U.S.-Mexican border. Furthermore, Tijuana is Baja California's biggest city, larger than San Diego to the north. Mexican IDUs are located mainly in cities such as Tijuana along the border with the United States (Badillo et al., 1998). Tijuana's red-light district seemed fertile ground to interview female street sex workers who might be IDUs sharing drug outfits and engaging in unprotected sex. It was important for this comparative investigation to determine:

- How knowledgeable and fearful were they of AIDS?
- What was the degree of their HIV-risk behavior, such as drug use and unprotected sex?
- How did they compare with street prostitutes in San Bernardino?

At the outset it seemed reasonable to assume that a higher HIV-positive rate existed among sex workers in Tijuana than in other large Mexican cities. High rates of IDU, unprotected sex with customers, HIV, and other STDs were likely to be found there among street sex workers.

Second, Tijuana was selected as a research setting because of its lawless reputation. Among the world's borderlands, the Mexican border with the United States has perhaps the most notorious reputation for vice, decadence, and unlawful activity. Cities such as Tijuana have achieved fame as playgrounds for pleasure-seeking Americans to drink, gamble, and buy sex (Martinez, 1994). Tijuana also has Baja California Norte's highest crime rate.

From 1940 to 1970 Tijuana rivaled Subic Bay in the Philippines, Shanghai, and the old Beacon Street of San Pedro, California, as a den of sex for sale, rowdy nightlife, drinking, and drugs. Like Subic Bay, American Naval and Marine personnel from San Diego flooded Tijuana on liberty. A massive sex industry spawned to meet the demand. In some bar stage shows donkeys reputedly had intercourse on stage with women.

In 1933, Tijuana was a sleepy little town of 13,000 inhabitants. Most of Tijuana's old money dates back to the Prohibition era, when many fortunes were made on gambling, brothels, and contraband. Poised along the U.S.-Mexican border, Tijuana today has over 2 million inhabitants, twice the size of San Diego. Although economic development has rehabilitated some of its downtown and new developments have sprung up (Millman, 1996; "San Diego Will Tell GOP," 1996), Tijuana is still the jumping-off point for thousands of would-be immigrants trying to make it to *el otro lado de la linea* ("the other side of the border") or to get jobs in Tijuana's own thriving economy (Millman, 1996; Sanchez, 1990). The service and business sector continue to represent the most important outlets for female employment in Tijuana, and education and employment among women in Tijuana is, on the average, higher than in all the rest of Mexico (Ojeda de la Peña and Rangel, 1996). Unemployment in Tijuana is dramatically smaller, and wages, while still abysmally low, are higher than in Mexico's heartland.

Baja California's high school graduation rate is the highest in Mexico, and university education is second only to Mexico City. There are twenty university campuses, think tanks, professional schools, and research centers between Tijuana and its companion city, Ensenada. Tijuana's better neighborhoods and strip malls are more like suburban Los Angeles than Mexico City. This is probably because of the intense cross-border visitation of Mexicans to Southern California. Ideas on what is au courant in Los Angeles, be it architecture, music, or gangs, quickly find their way to "TJ." However, the residential heart of Tijuana rises up on smoky-brown hills, where blocks lined with ramshackle houses are intersected by dirt streets without sewers, water hookups, indoor toilets, storm drainage, or gas service. These desperately poor *colónias* (neighborhoods) have exotic names such as Libertád (cradle of musician Carlos Santana), Obrera, El Florido, Matamoros, and La Miradór. The PRI party's liberal presidential candidate, Luis Donaldo Colosio Murrieta, was assassinated in a Tijuana slum in 1994.

Tijuana has a thriving underground economy, especially in drugs. It has made headlines recently as the site of gangland-style killings of top officials since the assassination of Colosio in March, 1994. An epidemic of drug-related, gangland-style murders has plagued Tijuana recently, prompting one U.S. prosecutor to compare the city to Chicago in the 1930s (O'Connor, 1996a,b).

Baja's drug wars, centered in Tijuana, have claimed the lives of a long line of drug kingpins, police officers, and government prosecutors. In February, 2000, Tijuana Police Chief Alfredo de la Torre Marquez was assassinated by gunmen who sprayed his Chevy Suburban with more than 100 bullets hitting him fifty-one times (Ellingwood and Perry, 2000). De la Torre was gunned down on the same street where one of his predecessors, Federico Benitez Lopez, was murdered in April 1994 in similar ambush fashion. Benitez's murder was thought to have been ordered by a drug cartel angered at his reformist ways. De La Torre's murder is reportedly linked to the notorious Tijuana drug cartel headed by the Arellano Felix brothers, Ramon, Benjamin, and Francisco (Ellingwood, 2000c). Reports also circulated in newspapers (Ellingwood, 2000d) that the assassinated Tijuana police chief had been cracking down in recent months on neighborhood drug dens and immigrant smugglers in the notorious zona norte, Tijuana's center for drugs and vice. Shortly after De La Torre's assassination, in May 2000, Mexican drug prosecutor Jose Patino Moreno, a ranking lawyer in the narcotics unit of the federal attorney general's office in Mexico City who was gathering evidence on the Arellano Felix drug gang in Tijuana, was tortured and murdered there along with two other anti-narcotics agents (Ellingwood, 2000b).

Based in Tijuana, the Arellano Felix cartel has become notorious as Mexico's bloodiest and most brutal drug empire. Authorities say that the cartel is headed by three Arellano brothers from Tijuana, all of whom have been in hiding since the 1993 assassination of Roman Catholic Cardinal Juan Jesùs Posadas Ocampo and six others at the Guadalajara airport. Ocampo is thought to have been mistakenly shot by an Arellano hit man who was trying to gun down one of the cartel's drug rivals. Members of the Arellano Felix cartel also have been blamed for the murders of scores of Mexican law enforcement officers. This gang was implicated in the execution-style slaying of twenty-one family members at a hacienda outside Ensenada in September 1998 (Ellingwood and Lightblau, 1998). Things are so hot for the Arellano Felix clan that they reportedly have moved much of their personnel away from Tijuana as law enforcement authorities have mounted crackdowns in the border city. The group's tentacles are now believed to have spread down the coast to Ensenada and east to Mexicali, Sonora (McDonnell, Ellingwood, and Tobar, 1998).

Tijuana coroner Gustavo Salazár believes that murders have increased because of a growth in local drug sales and consumption. He notes,

> There are well-known public officials who are assassinated for doing their jobs: fighting narcotics traffickers. Other men are killed because they want easy money and turn to drug trafficking. This is definitely on the rise in Tijuana. (O'Connor, 1996a, p. A1)

Mexican news accounts estimated that by mid-1999 the number of yearly murders statewide in Baja California Norte exceeded 300—most of them attributed to the drug trade. About 200 of them took place in Tijuana (Ellingwood, 1999).

Among *Tijuanenses,* confidence in police and judicial personnel is low due to corruption fueled by cartels dominating international drug trafficking, immigrant smuggling, and high-profile kidnappings. Veteran Tijuana prosecutor Jesús Romero Magaña was gunned down gangland-style in front of his home in August 1996, after he fired twenty-nine Baja California federal agents as part of a nationwide sweep of more than 737 members of Mexico's judicial police who were suspected of corruption, mainly involvement with drug rings (Sheridan and O'Connor, 1996). Three other prosecutors were also shot to death in Tijuana during 1996. Drug hits are made by people such as "El Kitty"—Everardo Arturo Paez Martinez, *"uno de los mejores gatilleros de los hermanos Arellano Felix, jefes del cartel de*

*Tijuana"* (one of the best trigger men of the Arellano Felix brothers, chiefs of the Tijuana cartel, who reside peacefully in the United States).

Rich Tijuana youths, "narco juniors," are enamored by the gangster glamour of the three Arellano Felix brothers, and many work as drug-smuggling "mules," and are often recruited by drug kingpins to carry out assassinations (O'Connor, 1996b). They drive new Corvettes, easily pay $45,000 bribes for release from jail, and fork over $29,000 for swank apartments (Solís, 1996). The most infamous street gang in Los Angeles, 18 Street, has established a base in Tijuana where, according to law enforcement officials, they pursue their criminal endeavors (Connell and Lopez, 1996).

What are the behavioral characteristics of FSWs in this environment, the face of which is hidden from ordinary tourists visiting Tijuana? Research for this book did not include venturing into the "tourist" bars. Instead, FSWs working in what is known as *zona norte* (on the north side of Tijuana) were interviewed. The *zona* is situated one block west of Avenida Revolucion at the intersection of First Street (Calle Uno) and Avenida Constitución. It is bounded by 1st Street on the south, Avenida Revolucion on the east, Avenida Baja California on the north, and "D" Street on the west. Avenidas Coahuilla and Baja California border the district. There are drastically fewer *norteamericanos* in this area than along the tourist strip of Avenida Revolucion. Perhaps they perceive it as too dangerous, or do not know where it is.

## *THE TIJUANA STREET INTERVIEW EXPERIENCE*

Señor Emílio Velásquez (whose father was an ex-mayor of Tijuana, and reputed to be one of the few honest ones) is the founding director of Organización SIDA Tijuana (Tijuana AIDS Organization; "SIDA"— Síndrome de Inmunodeficiencia Adquirida). This is Tijuana's only nongovernmental organization (NGO) engaged in HIV prevention, education, and hospice care for patients dying of AIDS. Señor Velásquez runs this operation out of his small coffeehouse in a back alley off Ave. Constitución. He has about 300 photographs of men dying of AIDS upstairs in his coffeehouse, a space that serves as a kind of hospice. Some pictures show dead men in coffins with candles all around and family members kneeling in prayer. There are pictures of Velásquez's station wagon with a coffin sticking out the back; he only has one coffin and keeps reusing it for dead AIDS victims.

Señor Velásquez introduced me to the first three street sex workers for interviews. They immediately recognized him the as the organizer of Vanguárdia de Mujeres Libres Maria Magdalena, a 107-member group of sex workers who spearheaded cessation of police harassment in Tijuana's red-light zone. Their lives are very difficult. Gay citizens, shunned in most of homophobic Mexico, have a niche in Tijuana, with clubs featuring female impersonators and one of Mexico's biggest annual gay pride marches. Some of the transvestites hug American boys and lift their wallets.

All interviews were confined to FSWs working the streets; none were interviewed in the sex bars, although there are numerous such establishments in the *zona*. A profusion of little bars in the red-light district cater to sex workers. FSWs entice customers to drink, and then make prostitution deals. Workers get *ficha* (a kind of kickback) off the bar tab. So do cab drivers and doormen. Sex acts are consummated in nearby hotels.

Typical "hooker bars" in the *zona* such as "La Carreta" and the "Chicago Club," are places where Mexican and American men come in, dance with the "bar girls," and go next door to a hotel for sex, which usually runs $10 for the room and $40 to 50 for "half-and-half," intercourse followed by oral sex. Some sex workers have hired their own security for hotels in which they work.

One Saturday night I counted 391 street prostitutes in a two-square-block area of the red-light district. This did not include women in the bars, of which there were probably twenty to thirty. A good portion of these sex workers, with no employment skills and low educational levels, fell into prostitution. Whatever the occupation, Tijuana seems to offer more opportunities for the poor than elsewhere in Mexico. It has a trickle-up economy, where the storied unemployment rate is allegedly only 1 percent, the envy of a nation (O'Connor, 1998).

After Sr. Velásquez introduced me to the first three subjects, I told each of them that I was a university professor, and gave each my business card. I said that I was a former heroin addict who had interviewed women like them in the Los Angeles area about how they felt about AIDS while prostituting and shooting heroin. I said that I was interviewing female sex workers in Tijuana to compare their responses with those of their counterparts on the streets of Southern

California. They were very interested in this cross-national approach, and seemed to feel an unspoken communion with their American sisters.

I asked each FSW if she would be willing to let me confidentially interview her, which would take about twenty minutes, for ten dollars (then about seventy-five pesos at the current rate of exchange). (I paid for the hotel or "crib" if these locales were used for interviews.) I questioned all Tijuana subjects in their own customary environment—on the street, in local restaurants, or in small five-dollar hotel rooms that cater to sex workers. I interviewed some in filthy "cribs" used exclusively for sex, located on second floors above commercial establishments. These one- to two-dollar rooms featured dirty mattresses on the floors, shared common toilets, used condoms, spit, and semen-littered floors.

Some respondents provided other subjects for interviews. At one point, I interviewed three women at one time in a little Chinese restaurant in the heart of the *zona*. We sipped sodas as they became more friendly and related freely their experiences as working prostitutes on the hard streets of their *distrito*. Interviews were conducted in Spanish, and the women spoke without inhibition. Almost every subject was extremely cooperative and open about the material bases of her everyday life. No reticence was encountered in answering blunt questions such as, *"¿Hace que los clientes usen condón o no?"* (Do you make your clients wear a condom?), or *"¿Chupa la verga?"* (Do you give head?).

A typical case was "Graciela," a solemn-mannered and graceful woman. "I am twenty-four years old," she told me in a more extended interview,

> I am from the state of Sinaloa. My father died when I was about a year old. I had older brothers and my mother supported us by doing housework for a family. My father's brother lived with us. I think he was about twenty-five years old. He slept in a room with my two brothers. I slept in a room with my mother. My uncle was a big man, maybe ninety to one hundred kilos. He paid my mother to stay with us, and his breath always smelled like alcohol.
>
> When I was little, maybe seven or eight years old, he used to feel my breasts, which were nothing then, and my vulva. Sometimes he would breath heavy and shoot stuff out of his penis.

I had my first menstrual period when I was about eleven years old. After that, when nobody was home, *mi tío* [uncle] would try to shove his penis into me. Gradually he stretched me, and sometimes it made me bleed. He said if I told anybody the *policía* would arrest me and put me in jail. So I let him do it. He would give me twenty pesos. I didn't go to school sometimes; I did the housework and cooking while my mother and my brothers were working. So I was always home with my uncle. When I was about sixteen he went off to work in California, and we moved to Tijuana. I missed the money he gave me. A neighbor girl said I could get more money by letting other *hombres* have intercourse with me. She worked below the church in *la zona*. So I went with her and she showed me what to do, how to get a license, what hotel to use, and what to do with customers. Business wasn't too good, but we made more doing this than at some *maquiladora* where you are overworked and underpaid. At first, my *cuñada* [girlfriend] said I wasn't charging enough, that I should charge more for each guy and that he should give me the money before he did it to me. Now I have enough money to live on, but barely.

I don't want to kiss any of them because their breath is so bad. This is purely work. The other girls showed me how to shorten up each time by holding a guy's testicles and moving around. The government requires a license, but my first [health] examination was a joke. The doctor just played around with me and gave me a certificate. When I told this to the other girls, they laughed. They said that was the easy way to a license. I don't have any other way to earn money.

Three years after these 1996 interviews, in 1999, I returned to Tijuana's *zona* and randomly interviewed ten more street workers. The responses were exactly the same as in 1996.

## *FSW INTERVIEWS IN CIUDAD JUÁREZ*

I chose Ciudad Juárez, state of Chihuahua, Mexico, as an interview site for several reasons. First, it has many similarities to Tijuana—border status, abundant crime, and drugs. Juárez is a huge border city, Chihuahua's largest municipality, with well over 2 million people—about 36 percent of the state's population. Like several other Mexican boarder cities, Juárez has a split personality. It is a booming manufacturing center with many U.S.-owned assembly plants *(maquiladoras)*. Juárez is also a city of criminal mayhem, known as a haven for *el negócio internacionál de las drogas* (international drug trade). Its red-light district sits inside a whirlwind, bordered by Begónias, Otumba, Degollado, Ocampo, and Mariscál streets just off the International Bridge, long a popular spot among military personnel from El Paso's 12,000-troop army base at Fort Bliss, and among male college students from Texas.

This city across the border from El Paso and home to one of Mexico's biggest narcotics cartels has a reputation for violence. The most perverse effect and the most important change that the drug market has introduced to Mexican society is the violence that drug trafficking breeds. As groups such as the Arellano Felix brothers in Tijuana battle to succeed Juárez drug kingpin Amado Carrillo Fuentes, who died a bizarre death in July 1997 after plastic surgery to hide his identity, the shootouts have increasingly spilled into the city's family restaurants, busy downtown streets, and quiet housing developments. Amado Carrillo Fuentes was legendary for his abilities to bully or coax Colombian drug traffickers into working with him. After his death on July 4, 1997, more than sixty-five people were killed in Ciudad Juárez during infighting among drug gangs (Sheridan, 1998a). The *narcotraficante* Carrillo Fuentes was known as *"El señor de los cielos"* (lord of the skies) because of his far-flung airplane fleet used in drug smuggling operations.

The result of the violence has been near-paranoia among Juárez residents. Gory contests for cartel dominance still make Juárez unsafe even for uninvolved residents who may get caught in the crossfire. In 1998 the rate of drug killings in Juárez was higher than it was in Miami during the Miami cocaine wars of the late 1970s. One local justice official in Ciudad Juárez states, "It's like the era of Al Capone. That's what we're living here" (Sheridan, 1998b, p. A1). In fact, in gubernatorial, state congressional, and city and county elections in Chihuahua, the number-one issue is public safety (Lopez, 1998). The worst moment for Juárez's image came in November 1999, when U.S. and Mexican drug enforcement agents descended on several ranches near the city, announcing that they had information about mass graves of victims slain by drug traffickers. U.S. officials spoke about possibly finding 100 to 300 bodies, though in the end, only nine corpses were unearthed (Sheridan, 2000). Nonetheless, it was yet another image nightmare for the bustling border city.

Hector Fuentes, a criminal justice MPA graduate student at University of Texas at El Paso and an El Paso County probation officer, accompanied me on a number of interviews with FSWs. Fuentes has lived in Juárez all his life and knows the city well.

The heart of the *zona* is filled with hundreds of female (and some transvestite) sex workers. This area parallels Juárez's main drag, Ave. Juárez. Most of the brothels are located near the main international bridge linking El Paso and Juárez.

A line of cabs waits on the Mexican side to take Americans to brothels to see or engage the women, for which the cabbies get a cut. These *taxistas* charge $3 to 5 U.S. The entire prostitution zone is about 1 km. square. Unless you keep your wallet in your front pocket here, it can be stolen. There are also some *masajes* (massage) parlors, such as Masajes Felina, Masajes Marisól, and Masajes Paradise. These are prostitution places. Some are very nice, offering not only "full-service" sex (anything the customer asks for, except sodomy), but also sauna, video, and a courtesy beverage. They advertise in the local Juárez newspaper.

In April 1998, Fuentes and I conducted interviews in the streets and in small brothels fronting the streets. This is a *real* red-light district: many tiny brothels actually had a red light hanging in front. Amateurs also work the street, and can be picked up and taken to a hotel room rented by the customer.

We conducted interviews in the streets with questionnaires laid out on the hoods of cars, on walls of buildings, and in a few bars. I hit mainly brothels—no bars, just rooms where the women solicit out of the front door facing the sidewalk. I'd sit on the couch in the "reception" area doing interviews, and in the women's bedrooms, for which I was never charged because of the "scientific" nature of my mission.

For regular customers in these brothels, there is usually a *nana*—an older woman—who comes into the room and hits up the customer for a few bucks for toilet paper and a condom. Her normal *propinita* (little tip) is a dollar. One Internet raconteur described Juárez prostitutes as ranging from "not bad/nice to dog shit." I found them mostly to be very pleasant in appearance. Some wore cocktail dresses, Lycra body suits, or midriff tops. I voluntarily paid each subject $20 U.S.

for interviews; they can charge more for sex (about $25 to $50 dollars) because of their proximity to the border.

The police presence in the area was heavy (bulletproof vests, belts full of bullets), and everybody seemed on good behavior. The women said the police never bothered them as long as they remained inside or very near the tiny street-front brothels.

All the subjects were licensed by the city and had weekly medical checks at the Centro de Salúd Familiár, a private medical clinic, which charged forty pesos (about $3.00) for each checkup. Most of the sex workers claimed to have blood tests for the presence of STDs once a month at a cost of eighty-five pesos. These women were more likely than those in other cities to perform less traditional sex, such as half-and-half. One very warm and friendly woman, "Amor," said she would "do anal," but *only* with a condom.

Women in Ciudad Juárez were more likely than those I interviewed in other Mexican cities to know someone in the prostitute community with AIDS. One pointed across the street to a dimly lit building and said that there was a former prostitute there dying of AIDS; that she was a *cocalero* (cocaine habitue).

I interviewed "Amor" who was forty-five years old with three children. Each night was a negotiation between hunger and dignity. A tiny woman in stiletto heels, zip-up top, and inch-long nails, she chatted with me out behind a parked car. She warmed up to me and took me to her room. I gave her ten dollars more and extended my conversation with her. I asked her where she was from and when she first started to have sex. She said she was born in San Juan del Rio, Durango, but came north to Ciudad Juárez to make money. She thought she began menstruating when she was about twelve,

> I used to masturbate every night, sometimes in the daytime when I would go outside to the toilet. My older sister saw this once; she said I was throwing myself away. She said I could be paid by guys to stick it into my vagina. She called this prostitution.
>
> One time, my cousin Ernesto came to visit us for a few days. He wasn't good-looking but he always had some money. He laid me on my cot and said he would give me fifty pesos if he could look at my vagina and feel my breasts. Without asking me, he shoved his hard penis into me. It hurt so bad I almost cried out. When he had shot out, he buttoned up his pants and said he

wasn't going to give me any money because I wasn't worth it. That's why the other girls in town said I should always be paid ahead of time. When I was twenty I went north to Ciudad Juárez. I met some girls there who worked in *la zona*. They said I could make quick money in the sex trade, more than in the *maquiladoras,* and I'd be my own boss. Lots of young *gabachos* (North Americans) come to Juárez to get drunk and buy prostitutes.

One time one of these *gringos* wanted his money back. He slapped me until I gave him the two hundred pesos back to him. The cops wouldn't do anything anyway; they don't care. I learned that if I pleased a guy by maybe putting his penis into my mouth first, he might even give me more pesos before he left. I don't mind what I'm doing for the money. I know that the high-toned office girls and some of the university girls do the same for money. The only difference is they have a regular salary. And what about wives? Don't they get married to be supported? Don't they give it to their husbands for pay? Someday I would like to write about this like you are. I wish I could write.

## FSW INTERVIEWS IN CIUDAD VICTORIA, TAMAULIPAS

I conducted interviews in Ciudad Victoria, capital of the state of Tamaulipas, for several reasons. First, because Tamaulipas state not only borders the United States (Nuevo Laredo, across from Laredo, Texas) but because it stretches south and east into a more tropical, drug-producing region of Mexico. Dr. Hector Lopez Gonzalez, director of health services for Tamaulipas state, told me during an interview in his Ciudad Victoria office that

> *Hay muchas lugares de siembra de drogas* [en Tamaulipas], *amapola y marijuana. Un gran cantidad de drogas se siembra en la montaña* (Tamaulipas State has many drug-growing places, poppies and marijuana. A great quantity of drugs is grown in the mountains). (Gonzales, personal interview, June 20, 1998)

In Ciudad Victoria, opiate use, introduced mainly by Chinese immigrants, began in the early twentieth century. It is believed that Chinese immigrants to Sinaloa and Sonora during the 1910s and 1920s were Mexico's first opium growers (Craig, 1989). A long-time resident and businesswoman recalled to me that as a child, when she accompanied her mother to the main public market in the city center, she regularly saw "old Chinese men smoking opium" (personal interview, June 18, 1998).

Six months after the assassination of PRI presidential candidate Donaldo Colosio in Tijuana, Jose Francisco Ruiz Massieu, president Zedillo's closest adviser and brother of Mexico's deputy attorney general in charge of antidrug trafficking, was gunned down on orders from Manuél Muñóz Rocha. Muñóz Rocha was a Tamaulipas PRI congressman, the state where Juan Garcia Abrego's drug trafficking was based. Abrego is now in prison in the United States on drug convictions. Police collusion with drug lords to protect drug shipments is so entrenched in Tamaulipas state that the Mexican army has been called in twice since 1989 to fire entire units of *federales*—federal judicial police. During a raid on the home and office of one police commander, the army found fifteen cars, a large stash of diamond-studded Rolex watches, and $5 million pesos. Another former police commander in Tamaulipas was found hiding a garment bag stuffed with U.S. $2.4 million in cash in the trunk of his car. He also paid more than $20 million to another antinarcotics elite *federale* to buy Garcia Abrego's protection (Paternostro, 1995).

Certain areas of Tamaulipas, such as the misty valley were Tomasenchale is situated, hang heavy with just the *feeling* that it is a big drug-providing place. Heavily armed state judicial police cruise the area in pickup trucks.

Another reason Ciudad Victoria was selected was because of a chance meeting with an excellent "guide" to the city's brothels, Dr. Russell Burrows. At seventy-two years old, he knew every bordello in the city, and enthusiastically led me on three days of intense interviewing. Like me, Burrows spoke fluent Spanish, and was thrilled to just sit around and chat with the prostitutes as I conducted face-to-face interviews with them. He gave me invaluable *entre* into the street-level sex service industry.

With Dr. Burrows' help, FSWs waited for interviews in working-class *cantinas* surrounding the inter-city bus depot. This area had lots of small "sex" *cantinas* and *hotelitos* where the FSWs take their clients. In these cantinas, FSWs will dance and hold you close; there is no cost for this, but customers usually buy them a beer or a soft drink. Clients proposition the FSWs in this manner, then they go across the street together to a small hotel for sex.

I interviewed six women in a *cantina* across from the bus station. Many small, working-class beer bars populated this area, all with prostitutes, no Americans in sight. For the sex act itself, they utilized small hotels in the area which charged ten pesos for the room. I paid each subject fifty pesos for an interview (about $6 U.S.).

A typical *cantina* respondent was twenty-seven-year-old "Elena" who was dressed in skintight denim jeans and had on indigo eyeliner; she was a bit drunk. She was very pretty, had a tattoo on her right upper breast, and enjoyed singing Mexican music along with the jukebox. Dr. Burrows' son, who had some emotional problems, was with Elena in the same *cantina* one night when Burrows found him and chased him out, waving a pistol. She remembered the incident, and reminded Dr. Burrows of it. Said Elena,

> This is work; I don't enjoy it. these men complain about their wives, work, their own loneliness. I'm a single mother supporting three children. I just keep my mind on the thirty to forty dollars a day I earn here. When it's slow, I can lose myself in the *cumbias* and *merengues,* and maybe dream a little. There's no danger in that.

Sex work is also conducted in small *hotelitos* such as "Hotel Ritz" (from whence comes the title of this book) which are strictly brothels. The fee for sex was about fifty pesos, around $6 U.S. All FSWs had official registration papers (Figure 4.1), a permanent card with photo, and the eight-day health card issued by the Hospitál Civíl. They paid thirty pesos a month for the registration card and health exam. The Hotel Ritz contained a small counter in the reception area, which sold and passed out keys to the rooms. The fee for the room was twenty-five pesos. The rooms were fairly clean, with a sheet on the double bed, and a toilet with no seat. The man at the reception desk, after I explained what the study was about, did not charge me for the room in which I conducted interviews. All of these women were sober, bright-eyed, and interested.

I also conducted interviews in another small Ciudad Victoria hotel-brothel, which was run by an eighty-year-old man who appeared to be the owner of the business. The cost for sex here was twenty pesos for the room and thirty pesos for the prostitute. Each room had a

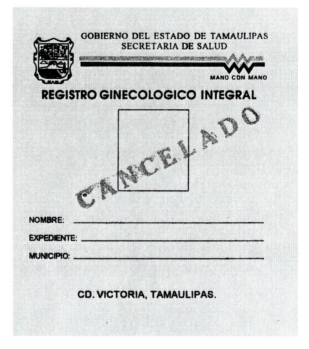

GOBIERNO DEL ESTADO DE TAMAULIPAS
SECRETARIA DE SALUD

MANO CON MANO

**REGISTRO GINECOLOGICO INTEGRAL**

CANCELADO

NOMBRE: _____

EXPEDIENTE: _____

MUNICIPIO: _____

**CD. VICTORIA, TAMAULIPAS.**

FIGURE 4.1. Prostitution license card. (*Source:* Tamaulipas State Department of Health)

bed with a dirty sheet, and a smelly toilet without a seat. These interviews were conducted at 11:00 a.m. on a weekday morning, and I observed only one client, a Mexican working-class man.

"Jesusita" led me back to her room. She seemed strong-willed and daring. I gave her extra money to tell me about how she got into the business. First she got pregnant. She bore a second child by an older man who was jailed on drug charges months after she gave birth. With her husband in jail and two babies to support, she went into prostitution out of desperation. "I'm twenty-four," she said,

> I grew up in Ciudad Valles, Tamaulipas. When I was about thirteen years old, my older brother would get into my bed almost every night. He would play with me until he got real hard and would gradually stretch me with his fingers and his penis. He had intercourse with me almost every night while my parents were sleeping. I expected it and I never thought it was wrong.

The other girls said their brothers did it to them, too. One girl said her brother came into her bed maybe twice a week and had intercourse with her and gave her extra money. I didn't mind. He said that's why girls and men are built the way they are. When I was about fifteen I moved here to Ciudad Victoria and lived in a small room with three other girls in back of a house out by the mall. We would go down and work the *cantinas* around the bus station. Sometimes we'd dress in short skirts with fishnet stockings, and not wear a bra. That would attract the men. I always had enough money.

Then I moved to this place because the rooms are cheaper than the hotels out by the bus station. Sometimes a guy with a lot of money gives me extra if I let him eat me out or I suck his penis and run my tongue around it. Some of the guys always want me instead of the other girls who work here.

I caught a disease from a boy who was vacationing with another boy. I had pus from my urethra and it burned when I urinated. I went to a doctor who gave me an injection and some tablets. He said I should get a license and that he would approve it. I got the same sickness another time, and it went into my abdomen [pelvic inflammatory disease?]. I had to be in bed for a week and couldn't work while the doctor gave me injections and tablets. He said I should insist that my customers wear rubbers for intercourse. So now I always make them use a condom. That's my rule. I don't need rubbers for my mouth except if I want to. I could earn some money, I would go to school to be a secretary. I know some of the girls at the university work on the side as prostitutes to make money. They make more because the men will pay more for "students." They think they are not professionals, or something. Understand? If I was a secretary then I could be a prostitute only when I needed extra money, and that would work out good.

My life is OK here. At least I eat and can take care of my kids.

The collective consciousness of a FSW.


## CUERNAVACA, MORELOS: ANOTHER INTERVIEW SITE

Finally, I conducted a set of Mexican interviews deeper in the republic's heartland, in Cuernavaca, capital of the state of Morelos, the summer home of Moctezuma, last of the Aztec kings. Morelos state has the fourth-highest rate of HIV/AIDS in Mexico (Vargas, 1998). Because of its pleasant climate on the direct route to Acapulco, Cuernavaca gets a heavy share of tourist trade, and has been known for years as a haven for American writers and other artists. However, it is a state political system noted for corruption ("Posición del PAN," 1998; Smith, 2001).

Cuernavaca seemed like a good place for interviews. Thirty years earlier the city's red-light district was brimming with prostitutes. In 1998, the state's governor, Jorge Carrillo Olea, was forced to resign from office on corruption charges. He was in the fourth year of a six-year term, and purportedly was related to the family of Amado Carrillo Fuentes, the recently deceased kingpin of Ciudad Juárez's international drug ring. Morelos today is so rife with kidnappings and corruption that the commander of the antikidnapping unit, Armando Martinez Salgado, was arrested in 1998 and convicted in 2001 on kidnapping and murder charges. After seventy-one years of one-party rule under PRI, only in 2000 did the first opposition party PAN (Partido Acción Nacionál) member accede to the governorship riding on the coattails of Vicente Fox.

Reliable "inside" ethnological information on local prostitution also prompted interviews in Cuernavaca. This "inside" information was provided by Aurélio Cruz-Valdéz, MD, chief of the Cancer Epidemiology Unit for the National Public Health Institute. In a "cold call" visit to his office located on the campus of the Universidád Auotónoma del Estado de Morelos, I asked him where I could find a lot of FSWs to interview.

He directed me to about six little *hotelitos* in Cuernavaca's downtown area, around the intersection of Matamoros and Arregón y León streets. As I arrived, prostitutes were spilling over from these small brothels, some hanging out in doorways, others in "reception" areas just inside, off the sidewalk. Pedestrians, including many women and schoolchildren, sauntered by, oblivious, and probably accustomed, to the sex business in progress around them. Almost all of the FSWs in these establishments were fairly young, attractive, of well-kept appearance, and very friendly after I apprised them of my research.

Interviews were conducted in the late afternoon and evening of July 13, 1998, during very hot weather. A drought was raging at the time throughout Mexico. Fires were devastating Mexico's countryside at the time, fueled by drought and El Niño. The Mexican government said that they were set intentionally. Loggers, ranchers, farmers, developers, drug traffickers, and soldiers in pursuit of Zapatista guerillas had all been looking to "clear" land for their own purposes (Russell, 1998).

The FSWs in these *hotelitos* charged a negotiable rate from fifty to seventy pesos and there was a twenty to thirty peso fee for the room. I paid each worker fifty pesos for an interview. Thirteen women worked in one of these establishments. The prostitute rooms were aligned around a nice courtyard, open to the air with tropical shade trees. Each room had two double beds, a mirror, a bare lightbulb, and an ubiquitous roll of toilet paper.

Typical of these subjects was "Daniela," a twenty-eight-year-old, handsome, dark-skinned Indian woman, who was short, thick, and muscular. She was hand feeding an *anciano* (old man) a bowl of chicken soup when I arrived. He had persistent diarrhea, and appeared severely debilitated. She said she was more afraid of *micróbios* that cause diarrhea than she was of contracting AIDS. She never had sex without a condom, though. She said she had a bad case of diarrhea two years ago that lasted two months. Daniela had one daughter and told me she wanted to leave the prostitution life in five years. She carried an official prostitute registration card and had an STD cursory exam every eleven days in a private clinic at a cost of forty pesos. She told me that prostitutes without a *boleto* (official registration card) worked the streets and the *zócalo,* but were subject to police pressure.

Daniela's parents, working-class Mexicans who previously had lived in the United States, knew what she did for a living, but did not approve. They always found themselves embroiled in fights over the prostitution life.

> I have been a prostitute since I was sixteen. I can get a guy to want me by dressing in short skirts, a tee shirt, and no bra to show my breasts. I started doing this for money, like the other girls. I'm from here. My father used to do it to me when he came home after drinking with other men. My mother knew about it and said she would tell the police. He said she could go ahead and they wouldn't have any money to live on.
>
> One time he brought another man with him to have sex with me. That guy gave me thirty pesos. The other girls showed me how to shorten up the job by pinching a guy's butt and moving

around. That way I can be paid for less time. The doctors who approved my license said I should buy some condoms and keep them ready to put on the guy. The doctor said I would have less chance of getting a disease. The health officials also gave me a book to read about diseases that prostitutes get, and how to prevent them. Some of us girls also were shown a film and got a lecture by the nurse over at the *hospital civil*. If I could save some money, I would have my teeth fixed and get out of this business; I have a daughter. Maybe I'd work in some office. I'm earning barely enough to live. I don't like what I'm doing; I would rather masturbate a guy, but I get only about half as much money for that.

A definite pattern of early childhood sexual abuse emerged from almost all of these interviews.

The "administration" of brothels such as this one in Cuernavaca where Daniela worked hold all the official sex work registration papers of the women who work in them. The documents are checked each month by public health officials, not police, who *revisan los papeles en la recepción* (check their papers at the registration desk). If papers are not in order, the brothel owners/operators are fined (a *multo*). Daniela was not afraid of contracting AIDS, and none of her fellow workers in the *hotelito* appeared to use drugs. They all required condoms. It has been proven that FSWs who do not use condoms are more at risk for HIV (Von Bargen et al., 1998).

# Chapter 5

# Findings: Comparing Mexican and San Bernardino Sex Workers

## *INTERVIEW RESEARCH QUESTIONS*

How *do* average Mexican street prostitutes compare with their San Bernardino, California, counterparts along the following variables?

- Background characteristics (age, education, marital status, number of children, duration of prostitution, and criminal history)
- HIV risk-related behavior, including:
  —Requiring client condom use and having frequent medical examinations to diagnose STDs and HIV
  —Knowledge and fear of HIV transmission
  —Awareness of other prostitutes in the area who are HIV positive or who have left the street trade because of AIDS fear
  —Likelihood of continuing prostitution if HIV positive
  —Injected and other drug-use patterns
- Client backgrounds, their sex act preferences, and attitudes toward AIDS
- Number of clients per day
- Fees charged

Answers to these questions could illuminate any cross-national differences in epidemiology, especially the incidence and prevalence of HIV infection and AIDS-risk behavior among Mexican street sex workers compared with their Southern California cohorts. This information is of immediate concern to improve the understanding of and to foster better public health among FSWs and their clientele on both sides of the border. The data obtained could provide solid fuel to launch policy recommendations to reform both antiprostitution and antidrug laws in the United States, where prostitution seems to be more of a police problem than one of public health. The findings may help clarify the sociology, economics, and current public policy setting of street prostitution in Mexico and in Southern California.

A world of difference exists between the street sex industry in Mexico and the United States. Through research for this book it was evident that Mexico is much more enlightened, progressive, and less puritanical than the United States in its policy approach to commercial sex. Why were the Mexican women so much less at risk for HIV than those in Southern California? The data herein provide some answers. Hypotheses will be suggested which might explain why leaders in these two countries have taken such divergent legal stances on street sex, and the results of such policies.

The sociocultural profile of Mexican female street sex workers is as follows:

- They are not alcoholics.
- They do not tend to be drug addicts. They generally are not "high" on crank (meth) or other drugs; they can't afford it.
- They are poor.
- They look at sex work as a job for survival, not as a means to earn money for drugs. Most American street prostitutes are under the influence, and many are on welfare/food stamps, using prostitution money to feed their drug habits. No such social safety net exists in Mexico. Women there prostitute for money for simple survival.
- Many tend to be immigrants where they work, usually from more rural, outlying areas.
- Sex workers who want business require customers to wear condoms.

### Similarities in Background Characteristics

Generally, there were no appreciable differences in marital status between the Mexican and American FSWs. Of the American sample, 15 percent were married; 12 percent of the Mexican women had husbands. Like the American sex workers, the Mexican women did not have "pimps" who lived off their earnings. The Mexican FSWs also were about the same age as their American counterparts: thirty-one years old, compared with age thirty for the Americans. Although the seventy-two San Bernardino IDU female street sex workers were a mixed race/ethnic group (47 percent Anglo, 43 percent Hispanic, 10 percent African American), almost all of the Mexican women (98 percent) were Hispanic. The Americans had been engaging in sex work for about five years, while the Mexicans had spent 6.5 years in the trade.

Like their American counterparts, every one of the 102 Mexican FSWs interviewed had heard of AIDS and were "very much" or "somewhat" afraid of contracting the disease. Although only three of the 102 Mexicans were IDUs, nine out of ten in both groups knew no one in the prostitute community who had stopped hooking or shooting drugs because of AIDS fear.

The customers of the American FSWs differed slightly from those of their Mexican peers. Among the American women, 56 percent said that most of their customers were "blue-collar types," while 41 percent of the Mexican FSWs reported that most of their clients were blue-collar. Whereas 19 percent of the Americans said that most of their "tricks" were businessmen, the Mexican FSWs categorized 8 percent of their clients as coming from this group. Whereas 3 percent of the San Bernardino FSWs said that their clients were "professionals," 8 percent of the Mexicans said they served primarily professionals. While 19 percent of the Americans said they provided services to "all kinds of johns," 43 percent of the Mexican FSWs said that socially, their customers were "all types." It is noteworthy that the Mexican women serviced few *Americanos* (11 percent American versus 89 percent Hispanics); in fact, almost no American "tricks" were observed in the red-light districts of any of the Mexican cities surveyed: the male pedestrians were overwhelmingly Mexican in Tijuana, Cuidad Juárez, Cuidad Victoria, and Cuernavaca.

## Differences Between Mexican and Southern California Female Street Sex Workers

Major differences exist between the Mexican and American prostitutes. The Mexicans sex workers were strikingly *more likely* than the American prostitutes to:

- Have monthly medical checkups (25 percent/13 percent; see Table 5.1)
- Be tested monthly for STDs as a legal requirement for engaging in prostitution (50 percent of Mexicans proven licensed versus 0 percent Americans)
- Have been tested for antibodies to HIV (72 percent/28 percent; see Table 5.2)
- Have tested positive for syphilis (2 percent/6 percent) and have had herpes genitalis on medical examination (3 percent/2 percent; see Table 5.3)
- Have sex with fewer clients per day (three versus eight for the Americans)
- Service only customers from their own race/ethnic group (89 percent/86 percent)
- Report that most customers want to use condoms (65 percent/8 percent), with a recent increase by clients in demanding this protection (46 percent/28 percent)
- Require condom use, including for fellatio (92 percent/14 percent; see Table 5.4)
- Have condoms in their possession (55 percent/0 percent; see Table 5.4)
- Have dependent children (the Mexicans about two each; the Americans one)
- Charge less for penis-vaginal intercourse ($7 versus $30 charged by the Americans)
- (If IDU) purchase narcotic injection paraphernalia legally (100 percent no)

TABLE 5.1. Frequency of Medical Checkups

| | Mexicans (%) ($n = 102$) | Americans (%) ($n = 72$) |
|---|---|---|
| Weekly | 56 | 0 |
| Every two weeks | 4 | 6 |
| Every three weeks | 2 | 6 |
| Monthly | 25 | 13 |
| Now and then or never | 13 | 75 |

TABLE 5.2. HIV Testing, Drug Use, and Crime Patterns of All Mexican and San Bernardino Street FSW Subjects

| | Mexicans (n = 102) | Americans (n = 72) |
|---|---|---|
| Ever been tested for HIV? | 73 (72%) | 20 (28%) |
| Keep working the streets if HIV+? | 8 (8 %) | 36 (50%) |
| Under influence of heroin, cocaine, methamphet- amine, or alcohol at interview | 3 (12%) | 72 (100%) |
| Ever used IV drugs? | 3 (12%) | 72 (100%) |
| How much do you spend a day on IV drugs? | $20 | $170 |
| Do you have husband/boyfriend who uses IV drugs? | 3 (3%) | 58 (81%) |
| Ever been arrested for a crime? | 40 (39%) | 68 (94%) |
| Ever been convicted of a crime? | 32 (31%) | 62 (86%) |
| Ever done time in jail/prison? | 32 (32%) | 60 (83%) |
| Do more clients bring up the subject of AIDS lately? | 28 (27%) | 60 (83%) |

TABLE 5.3. Number Testing Positive for Syphilis, Gonorrhea, Herpes Genitalis, or HIV

| | Mexicans (n = 102) | Americans (n = 72) |
|---|---|---|
| Syphilis | 2 (2%) | 4 (6%) |
| Gonorrhea | 15 (15%) | 36 (50%) |
| Herpes genitalis | 3 (3%) | 1 (2%) |
| HIV | 0 | 2 (3%) |

TABLE 5.4. Precautions with Customers to Avoid Sexually Transmitted Disease

| | Mexicans (n = 102) | Americans (n = 72) |
|---|---|---|
| Require customers wear a condom | 94 (92%) | 11 (14%) |
| Suggest customers wear a condom | 8 (8%) | 37 (51%) |
| Inspect customer's penis for signs of STD | 25 (25%) | 6 (8%) |
| Wipe/wash off customer's penis | 2 (2%) | 4 (6%) |
| No precautions taken | 0 | 18 (25%) |
| Do you have any condoms on you now? | 56 (55%) | 0 |

On the other hand, the Mexican FSWs were less likely than their American cohorts to:

- Be under the influence of heroin, cocaine, methamphetamines, or alcohol at interview (12 percent/100 percent; see Table 5.2)
- Ever use IV drugs (12 percent/100 percent; see Table 5.2) or spend over $30 a day on drugs ($20 a day for each of the three Mexican IDUs versus $170/day for American IDUs; see Table 5.2)
- Have IDU husbands/boyfriends (see Table 5.2)
- Keep working the streets if she became HIV positive (8 percent/ 50 percent; see Table 5.2)
- (For those tested) Permit over four months to elapse between HIV tests (5/13, 39 percent versus 20/20, 100 percent)*
- Report being HIV positive (0 versus 3 percent) or to have had gonorrhea (15 percent versus 50 percent; see Table 5.3)
- Be arrested (39 percent versus 94 percent), convicted (31 percent versus 86 percent), or incarcerated for crimes (32 percent versus 83 percent; see Table 5.2)
- Know that the HIV is transmitted by *both* unprotected sex and injecting drugs (41 percent versus 83 percent; see Table 5.6)
- Engage in combined penis-vaginal intercourse and fellatio ("half-and-half," 31 percent/75 percent) or sodomy (1 percent/ 8 percent; see Table 5.5)
- Respond that over 25 percent of their customers were afraid of being infected with HIV by a sex worker (0 percent/83 percent)
- Report that customers do not like to use condoms (8 percent/64 percent)
- Recall that more clients were bringing up the subject of AIDS lately (27 percent/83 percent; see Table 5.2)
- Be high school graduates (seventh grade was the mean for the Mexicans; eleventh for the Americans)
- Be informed about HIV transmission (see Table 5.6)
- Service more than three clients a day

---

*Monthly tests for other STDs are mandatory for legal prostitution licenses in most of Mexico.

TABLE 5.5. Type of Sex Customers Want Most Frequently

|  | Mexicans (n = 102) | Americans (n = 72) |
|---|---|---|
| Penis-vaginal intercourse only | 72 (70%) | 8 (11%) |
| Fellatio | 25 (24%) | 16 (22%) |
| Sodomy | 1 (1%) | 6 (8%) |
| Cunnilingus | 8 (8%) | 2 (3%) |
| Masturbation | 5 (5%) | 0 |
| Intercourse and fellatio ("half & half") | 32 (31%) | 54 (75%) |

TABLE 5.6. Respondents' Understanding of AIDS Transmission

|  | Mexicans (n = 102) | Americans (n = 72) |
|---|---|---|
| Unprotected sex only | 56 (55%) | 5 (7%) |
| Injecting drugs only | 4 (4%) | 6 (8%) |
| Unprotected sex *and* IV drugs | 42 (41%) | 60 (83%) |
| Don't know | 0 | 0 |

## *ANALYSIS AND DISCUSSION*

These data clearly show that in a variety of ways, the Mexican prostitutes were less exposed to HIV infection than American IDU street sex workers. A further distinguishing dimension is, unlike their American cohorts, only three Mexicans (12 percent) were IDUs. In general, the Mexican women took more precautions to prevent infection with HIV and other STDs. Why?

### *Legal Prostitution and Mandatory Medical Examinations in Mexico*

Prostitution is legal in most Mexican states (it is a state option). As in some other nations, FSWs have been demanding the right to organize into unions. A recent article in Mexico City's leading daily newspaper noted, "In Latin America sex workers are asking that their work be recognized as a legitimate job, and that they should have the right to organize" (*Excelsiór*, 1998).

In Mexico, prostitutes can only get a license if they have a negative health examination. Fifty percent (13/26) of the women interviewed in Tijuana could produce these city health licenses, which display a woman's official photograph, age, address, file number, and other pertinent data. This health licensing requirement reflected more frequent medical examinations (see Table 5.2). The data gathered in these studies indicate that the Mexican sex workers were less likely than their American cohorts to have had HIV or gonorrhea (see Tables 5.2; 5.3). Other reports show that HIV postitive status among the female prostitution population in Tijuana is about 1 percent (Velasco-Hernandez, 1997). To acquire and maintain licenses, sex workers must pay eighty-five pesos ($11.50) a month and must be checked each month for:

- *sifilís*
- *gonorrea*
- *candidiasis*
- *herpes genitalis* (examined; no test)
- *tricomoníasis*
- *chancro blando* (chancroid)

To be licensed, Tijuana sex workers must be tested every four months for HIV with an enzyme-linked immunosorbent assay (ELISA) and, if positive, confirmed by a Western Blot. Antibody results apparently are provided to the licensing unit. These regulations eventuate in less HIV exposure, and could partially account for less fear of AIDS among Mexican clients` compared with American clients (see Table 5.2).

### Sexual Precautions to Reduce HIV Exposure Risk

All of the Mexican women in this study took *some* precautions with customers to prevent the spread of HIV and other STDs. Even 89 percent of Ivory Coast FSWs reported condom use in 1997 (Ghys et al., 1998), and, reportedly, 100 percent of foreign FSWs in Japan require condom use (Sankary et al. 1998). *One-fourth (25 percent) of American FSWs took no precautions* (see Table 5.4). Seventy-seven percent of the Mexican prostitutes said that they required condom use. They did not seem afraid of losing clients if they insisted on condoms. These findings are contrary to those in a study of Cuidad Juárez prostitutes, where erratic condom use was indicated by many of the women. A subjects in this investigation reported,

> Most tricks don't like to use condoms. If I don't have one, the hell with it . . . Mexican men don't like using it, it hurts their manhood. They say they can't please a women [sic] with that. Anglo men are smarter to that effect . . . man, they're married . . . they ought to use a rubber . . . some men do not care. (Deren et al., 1997, p. 209)

Whereas studies have reported that most American street prostitutes require clients to use condoms, even for fellatio (Symanski, 1981; Zausner, 1986), in this study, 14 percent of the American women reported that they required condom use (see Table 5.4). (Both clients and sex workers appear to be whistling in the dark.) While none of the American women who said they required condom use could produce a condom during the interviews, almost all (85 percent) of the Mexicans could do so. A Mexican prostitute was three times more likely as an American to inspect or wash her customer's penis before intercourse or fellatio (see Table 5.4).

In sum, generally all the Mexican sex workers took more precautions to reduce HIV risk exposure than the American IDU street sex workers. Without exception, the Mexican women said that if they did not want to contract AIDS, their most important precaution would be "*protegerme*—protect myself [by requiring condom use]."

As another FSW said, "I protect myself *and* them." When probed about what they would do if a client insisted on intercourse without a condom, typical responses were,

> "I always use a condom. *Si no, no me voy*" (if they won't use a condom, I won't have sex with them).

> "If they want sex without a condom, I'll talk to them, and try to convince them that it's best for them and their family, and for me, if they use protection. Then they go along with it."

> "I always put the condom on for them. That makes it easier."

Findings on required condom use among Tijuana FSWs confirm those of another investigation of sex workers there in 1996, in which prostitutes working in clubs, bars, and on the street were interviewed. "Women," said this study, "reported that they almost always use a condom with their clients . . ." (Rosas, Rangel, and Diaz, 1996, p. 42).

### Comparative Drug Use Behavior

All seventy-two of the San Bernardino sex workers interviewed were heroin addicts out hooking primarily for drug money. Their individual heroin habits ranged between $100 and $350 day, with a mean of $200. They injected heroin between four and six times daily. The seventy-two-member sample spent a combined $15,000 *daily* on Mexican "black tar" and powdered Mexican brown heroin, sometimes laced with cocaine in a "speedball." Although the American study was confined to IDUs, 90 percent of the American women approached were obviously under the influence of mind-altering drugs. When asked if they would like to clean up (get off heroin), most said yes. Responses included,

"Of course."

"Yes. I want to get off heroin more than the streets."

"Not really. I can't."

"My body won't work without heroin. I hurt and get cramps."

"It's so easy to make money [hooking]."

"Been using for fifteen years. I've hardly ever been clean, except in jail."

"I hook to shoot dope and shoot dope to hook."

This study indicates that the Mexican FSWs randomly interviewed presented an entirely different picture: substantially less HIV risk-related behavior. As for drug use, compared to the San Bernardino women, the Mexican FSWs were "choir girls" (Table 5.2). About the most drugs they used, except for a few IDUs in Tijuana, was *mari-*

*juana, a veces* (marijuana, once in a while) and *cerveza* (beer). This differs from findings in another study of twenty Mexican prostitutes conducted in Cuidad Juárez, which revealed more IDU than found in this study (Deren et. al., 1997). However, it is generally believed among researchers, that in Mexico, FSWs have reduced opportunities for hard drug abuse and are heavily stigmatized for such behavior (Mondragon et al., 1998). In Mexico's main HIV/AIDS surveillance study, only 0.8 percent of the female population were identified as IDUs (Rodríguez, Ruiz-Badillo, et al., 1998). Other international studies of FSWs, such as one conducted in Bangladesh among 205 women near a ferry and train station showed virtually *no* IDU (Mahmud et al., 1998).

In the Mexican subjects there were no stigmata of IDU: intravenous puncture wounds in the arms or on the backs of hands ("marks," "tracks"); pupillary dilation or constriction; somnolence of narcotic intoxication, or the agitation characteristic of amphetamine or cocaine use; rarely, the odor of alcohol on the breath.

Mexican FSWs, especially in Tijuana and Cuidad Juárez, seemed to exist in the eye a criminal hurricane of drug murders, heroin/cocaine/methamphetamine/marijuana smuggling, police and judicial corruption, and the average citizen's pervasive fear of lawlessness. *Mexico es un lugar de tránsito de droga y productór de drogas* (Mexico is a drug transshipment and production nation).

Of the three Mexican subjects (12 percent) who reported IDU, one injected heroin, the other two methamphetamines. The subject who injected pure methamphetamine was a transvestite in effective female disguise. He said that his clients liked to be penetrated rectally by a man dressed as a woman.

Sample bias and geographic locale may account for the low IDU rate observed in the Mexican sample. In other *bárrios* in Tijuana, or especially other border cities, IDU may be more prevalent among sex workers. In Mexicali, Baja California Norte, for example, which is about 100 miles east of Tijuana, there is a prostitution *zona* known as Palaco where IDU reportedly is high among female sex workers (Velásquez, H., personal communication). There, an average dose of heroin costs $3.00 (compared with $25-$50/dose in San Bernardino).

Legalized prostitution in Mexico and low rates of IDU among the Mexican sex workers interviewed seem to account for less criminal involvement than their American IDU cohorts (see Tables 5.2 and 5.6).

The most "time" done by the Mexican women ranged from thirty minutes to a maximum of thirty-six hours in jail, usually for being out on the street or not having a license. The Mexicans were not pursued by police for violation of antiprostitution and antinarcotic laws. Drug dependence and the need for drug money did not propel them, as it did their San Bernardino cohorts, to commit crimes such as forgery and property theft, nor did they have to prostitute for drug money.

Nine out of ten American IDUs interviewed shared their outfits with other addicts—51 percent with at least four others, 8 percent with ten or more addicts (Bellis, 1990). The bleak assessment: this high sharing rate is probably due to scarcity of legal outfits.

Like their American sisters, none of the three Mexican IDUs had modified her needle-sharing practices because she was afraid of AIDS: all shared their outfits with one another (but none with more than two others). However, their injection equipment could be purchased without prescription in Tijuana's hundreds of *farmacias*.

In the United States, nonprescription sales and possession of outfits are illegal. Moreover, disposable needles purloined by American addicts are designed for single use. (In the old days, addicts used eyedroppers, baby pacifiers, and stainless steel hypodermic needles that could be boiled and sharpened.) Reuse of today's disposable syringes causes needles to become dull and to break; outfits become scarce, and IDUs end up sharing when they need a fast shot to overcome the craving of withdrawal. Infinitely less sharing occurs among Tijuana's few IDU female street sex workers, who have easier access to supplies of disposable syringes *(jeringas)* and needles *(agujas)*.

## Comparative Sociology and Economics of Street Sex Work in Mexico and the United States

The sociology and economics of street sex work in Mexico are different from San Bernardino. Mexican FSWs are poorer and less involved in drugs than their American counterparts, often permanently excluded from participating in mainstream labor market occupations. They look upon their occupation as strictly a job, not a way to finance a drug habit.

Several conditions may explain why the Mexican FSWs used fewer illegal drugs than the American subjects interviewed. First is the emphasis on social networks and families in Mexico, which provide more social support and nurture. There is less stress. Mexico has more insulating family structures, socially enforced safe behavior, and less risky lifestyles than Americans. Generally, Mexican women are less likely to smoke, drink, and use drugs than American women. Interestingly, few Mexican-American women abuse alcohol or illegal drugs. Although 75 percent of Mexican immigrant women do not drink, only 36 percent of American women abstain from alcohol (Nazario, 1999). Drugs still carry a stigma in Mexico. In Mexico, especially in rural areas, women who drink or use illegal drugs are considered "loose." The Mexican women interviewed appeared poor, most of them were from more rural areas in Mexico, and were naive about drugs.

Unlike some American prostitutes, Mexican prostitutes have no social welfare safety net upon which to fall. Prostitution is their sole source of support. At a maximum income of $20 a day from prostitution *they can't afford drugs.*

The American IDU sex workers paid living expenses through public assistance such as Temporary Assistance for Needy Families (TANF), housing subsidies, and with food stamps while shooting up their prostitution earnings (at an average rate of $170 a day). No such luxury for the Mexican sex worker: to eat, she must keep her nose to the grindstone and not mess around with drugs.

Injected drugs produced in Mexico (*goma*—black tar heroin, or Mexican brown powdered heroin; methamphetamine) are used infrequently there, but are destined for shipment to the world's largest drug market: the United States.

That the Mexican sex workers served fewer clients per day than their American counterparts (3/8) may be due to more intense competition for customers in red-light districts. Tijuana was a good example. With 300 prostitutes working a one-square-block area and numerous others in sex bars, the competition is obvious. The supply of Tijuana sex workers in this area seemed to far outweigh the demand. Poverty could explain the oversupply of prostitutes.

### Knowledge and Fear of AIDS

Like the San Bernardino prostitutes, all of the Mexican subjects knew about AIDS, probably because of their occupation. In a study of AIDS knowledge among *rural* women in Mexico, 43 percent had heard of the disease (Velóz, Coeto, and Villegas, 1998). In this study, 83 percent of the American subjects mentioned both unprotected sex and injecting drugs as the main modes of HIV transmission; 41 percent of the Mexican sex workers knew this relationship (see Table 5.6). HIV education/prevention outreach efforts into the sex worker communities has been more intensive in the United States than in Mexico. The head of the Mexican Social Security Hospital's AIDS unit in Mexicali said that his agency does not conduct HIV prevention/education programs in the schools, among drug users, or within the sex worker communities (Ontiveros, personal interview, 1995).

Were the FSWs afraid of contracting AIDS? All seventy-two American FSWs were "very much" or "somewhat" afraid of HIV transmission. Twenty-one FSWs (58 percent) said that other IDU street prostitutes they knew were afraid of AIDS. Typical comments on fear of AIDS included:

> "Shit yes, 'bro."

> "Yea, I'm concerned, until I stick the needle in. When I'm hurting, dope's the only thing on my mind."

> "I'm afraid of AIDS, out hooking and shooting dope. I know it's really dangerous."

> "My parents know what I'm doing, and they're worried about me gettin' it.

> "I'm afraid of AIDS, but I've got a drug problem. Drugs drive me. If it weren't for heroin, I wouldn't be out here doin' this. Dope pushes everything else out of my mind."

Five times as many San Bernardino prostitutes than Mexicans would keep working the streets if they had AIDS (see Table 5.2). Since all of the American subjects were IDUs (with staggering costs for heroin habits), the necessity of money for drugs probably drove their choice to keep prostituting in the face of AIDS. Typical of the American "Bonnie and Clyde" comments on continuing to prostitute with AIDS was, "Baby, my boyfriend and I'd go out in a blaze of glory, shootin' dope and robbin' banks!" Other individuals noted,

"I can't stop using."

"Yea, I'd die anyhow I'd probably keep hooking and using."

"I'm making good money."

"I'd go deeper into the spoon [heroin cooker]. Depressed. I wouldn't commit suicide, though, because I'd want to fix to-morrow."

"Yes, figure I'd die anyhow."

"Sure . . . what the hell."

The Mexican nonaddicts probably found it easier to drop out of the prostitution lifestyle if they became HIV positive because they were not compelled by the drive of addiction. Typical of their open-ended responses to continued prostitution if diagnosed with AIDS was, "*Seguro* (sure), I'd quit prostitution and get another kind of job."

### Client Sexual Preferences and Attitudes Toward AIDS

The most popular sex act for San Bernardino clients was a combi-nation of penis-vaginal intercourse and fellatio (75 percent), but 70 per-cent of Mexican males wanted plain, penis-vaginal intercourse (see Table 5.5), *sexo normál*.

Although more Mexican customers than Americans wanted to use condoms, they appeared less afraid of HIV infection. Both the Mexi-can and American FSWs observed that there has been a recent increase in the number of customers bringing up AIDS, but fewer of the clients in Tijuana broached the subject (see Table 5.2). The Mexican women reported that 25 percent of their clients expressed some fear of HIV infection from a sex worker; the American women said that 85 per-cent of their customers mentioned something about this. Open-ended responses from the San Bernardino addict-prostitutes included,

"Nine out of ten [new] tricks ask me if I'm afraid of AIDS."

"Most of them bring up the subject of AIDS. They ask me if I'm afraid of catching it, and what I do about it."

"Yes, they'll ask something about me being 'clean.'"

"More johns bring it up lately. They ask me if I take good care of myself."

However, the general feeling among the American women was that the compulsive drive for sex overrode customers' AIDS fear. "A guy's brains are in his dick," replied one respondent, "why else would these assholes be out here?"

Paradoxically, the better-educated American clients were less likely than Mexican men to use condoms during intercourse. One American IDU street sex worker told me that almost all of the new tricks asked her if she was afraid of AIDS. Typical of the responses of Mexican sex workers were:

"If a customer asks if I'm clean, or brings up the subject of AIDS, I show him my *boleto* (license) listing the results of my health exams, and that's it!"

"If they ask, I show them my card—*mi registro* (registration)."

"*Muestro la tarjeta* (I show them my card)."

# Chapter 6

# Summary, Recommendations, and Conclusions

Mexican FSWs have contained the spread of HIV infection and STDs by (1) avoiding IDU; (2) careful precautions with clients; and (3) legal prostitution with mandatory medical examinations and testing for STDs and HIV. Mexico presents a clear-headed view of prostitution. It is tolerated and controlled, not by arrests and marginalizing, but by zoning, licensing, and periodic examination of FSWs for STDs. The Mexican prostitutes in this study, although poor and working in head-to-head competition, face a less bleak health future than the American FSWs interviewed in San Bernardino.

## *RECOMMENDATIONS FOR MEXICAN FSWs*

What, finally, can be gleaned from interviews with Mexican and American prostitutes? For *Mexican* FSWs, three recommendations stand out to keep spread of STDs and HIV under control:

### 1. Reduce or eliminate prostitute health license fees.

One problem with the Mexican FSW license fee is that it acts as a disincentive to regular STD testing. Only half (this means half *had* one) of the Mexicans interviewed could produce their health licenses. If the licenses were free, maybe more Mexican FSWs would obtain them, eventuating in more regular health exams and even lower STD rates.

Public policies have paradoxical effects, sometimes called "unintended consequences" (Dye, 1992). Mandatory testing for STDs among FSWs in Athens, Greece, has produced a two-tier system of registered and nonregistered prostitutes, the latter having little access to health care. Greece has the strictest prostitution regulations in Europe, requiring mandatory medical screening twice a week. This impels most FSWs there to avoid registration. All health care facilities and HIV prevention activities for Greek prostitutes are limited to those who are registered. This is ineffective control: in Athens about 400 women are registered, while an estimated 5,000 more prostitutes are unregistered. These official figures are underestimated in a city of 4 million.

In the United States, there should be no penalties or fees associated with STD testing among FSWs.

## 2. Introduce an intensive STD prevention/education campaign in Mexican primary and secondary schools, and HIV testing/prevention/education street outreach among homosexual/bisexual males, drug users, and sex workers.

While 76 percent of Mexican adolescents know how HIV is transmitted, only 15 percent know how to prevent transmission; girls are less likely than boys to know about modes of transmission (Cruz-Valdez et al., 1998).

With the poor track record of the Mexican federal government in HIV seroprevalence studies and AIDS prevention/education, nongovernmental organizations (NGOs) such as Organizacion SIDA Tijuana should be utilized to conduct these programs (Velásquez, E., personal communication, 1996; Hartigan, 1994). Mexican governments and private businesses should partner with NGOs to conduct seroprevalence studies, care for those patients with AIDS-opportunistic illnesses, and prevent HIV infection through early education.

If street-based and other specialized education efforts were intensified in Mexico among at-risk groups such as sex workers, with careful evaluations of behavioral outcomes and epidemiologic data collection, HIV/AIDS and HCV infections might be reduced to even lower levels.

## 3. Continue legalized prostitution in controlled settings or *zonas*.

*A la zona* ("to the prostitute district!") has long been the destination for a "night out" for Mexican men. It does not make it right, but that's the way it is. These zones of tolerance probably do reduce crime, protect public health, and greatly reduce economic costs associated with crime and illness. Scientific research proves that licensed prostitutes worldwide who operate in restricted zones have lower HIV infection rates than those outside these locales. For example, in Germany, *no* licensed prostitutes operating in legal zones who were tested were HIV positive (Smith, 1986), while under Bombay's unlicensed system, 47 percent were HIV positive (Geeta, Lindan, and Hudes, 1995).

## RECOMMENDATIONS FOR AMERICAN FSWs

For *American* heroin-addicted FSWs (and heroin addicts generally), the following recommendations should be considered:

### 1. Better HIV/AIDS/STD prevention and treatment programs.

The major factors in STD and HIV transmission such as IDU, prostitution, and risk discounting are hard to counteract. Would HIV-prevention education work among American addict-FSWs? Some studies among in- and out-of-treatment IDUs show less sharing of injection paraphernalia after community outreach intervention/education programs (Colón, et al., 1995; McAuliffe et al., 1987; Watters, 1987; Wiebel et. al., 1996). Other studies are more skeptical of the effectiveness of prevention education among addicts (De Jarlais and Friedman, 1988; Fineberg, 1988; Flynn et al., 1987; Bellis, 1983; 1990). Nonetheless, targeted intervention/education programs on condom use and clean injection paraphernalia should be expanded. More frequent condom use by FSWs is positively associated with exposure to a targeted intervention program (Ghys et al., 1998).

Can American IDU female street prostitutes, who hook for drug money, change their behavior in time to prevent HIV or HCV infections? Can they be relied upon to clean their paraphernalia for re-use with bleach or alcohol, using clean rinse water, when they are sick during withdrawal and need a fix? Can one of the most compulsive of human behaviors—narcotic addiction—be changed by simply *telling* addict-prostitutes to think and behave rationally just when they are most vulnerable? The dreadful irony is that the severe discomfort of narcotic withdrawal is the strong motivator to take risks (Stein, 1993; Bellis, 1983).

For HIV control programs to be effective among FSWs, the cooperation of sex workers, skilled, well-paid staff with sympathetic attitudes, and convenient locations for prostitutes are all required. Outreach is essential.

Occasional female prostitutes, transsexuals, transvestites, and male prostitutes are harder to reach with HIV-prevention strategies. STD prevention/education programs must be free of charge and must build links with existing services such as addiction treatment, social support and counseling, and should cooperate with needle exchange and methadone maintenance clinics.

Postintervention evaluation is necessary in any HIV and HCV control program among FSWs. Control group designs are best, but it is difficult to find a representative sample in this often criminalized and stigmatized group. Understandably, many FSWs who are IDUs do not like to be interviewed by "lames" with long-winded, standardized questionnaires, and they do not like to be treated as research subjects.

### 2. *Free* methadone maintenance for heroin addicts, especially addict prostitutes.

Most treatment professionals say that long-term narcotic addiction treatment works at least as well as long-term treatment for other chronic diseases, such as diabetes, dramatically reduces illicit drug abuse, and is much more effective than jail or prison. One-year relapse rates for heroin addiction are about 50 to 80 percent. Private residential drug-treatment programs range from $4,400 to $6,800 for one client per year; methadone maintenance averages about $2,000 a year. Keeping one drug addict in prison costs about $30,000 per year. Federal, state, and local governments should increasingly fund addiction treatment. It is an undisputed fact that narcotic addiction treatment, especially methadone maintenance, prevents HIV infection among IDUs (Bellis, 1993; also see Bellis in Sorensen and Copeland, 2000). Free methadone maintenance should be made available immediately to all addicts who request it. Methadone has been available only under strict federal and state laws and licensing procedures which control dosage. These controls should be relaxed, and physicians allowed to dispense methadone upon prescription to America's estimated

600,000 heroin addicts. Dosage levels should be left to physicians, based on individual cases. The federal government spends only 20 percent of the nation's $20 billion drug-control budget to treat addicts (Neergaard, 1998). Unfortunately, where IDUs are concerned, there are far fewer free patient slots in drug abuse treatment programs than there are drug injectors (Friedman and Lipton, 1991).

Methadone maintenance works. Methadone hydrochloride (adolphine, dolophine, adanon, amidone, physeptone, althose, miadon, butalgin, diadone, polimadone) is a synthetic substitute for heroin. It was first synthesized by the German firm I.G. Farben in 1941 when the Nazi regime's organic opium supplies dried up on the Turkish front. Methadone maintenance is the dispensing of oral methadone to replace dependence on heroin, and has been used in the United States in treatment of opioid dependence for over fifty years. Although the drug is as addictive as heroin, it is effective and safe in long-term administration. Herman Göering reportedly flew aircraft while taking it.

An adequate, individualized daily dose of methadone (60-200 mg) eliminates narcotic drug craving, prevents the onset of withdrawal, and blocks (through opiate cross-tolerance) the effects of typical other opiates, such as heroin or morphine. When ingested by an addict, the drug has the same effects as heroin, though its duration of effect is much longer (twenty-four hours compared with six hours for heroin). By 1970, most knowledgeable clinicians agreed that methadone maintenance was "the preferred treatment for long-established heroin addiction" (Goldstein, 1970, p. 311). Dr. Vincent Dole, the leading proponent (with his late wife, Dr. Marie Nyswander) of methadone maintenance for over forty years, is adamant in his belief that this heroin control treatment remains the best one in normalizing the functioning of injecting heroin users (Dole and Nyswander, 1965; Dole, 1966, 1967, 1976, 1997). Other clinical research (Bellis, 1993) supports Dole.

Efficacy of methadone maintenance treatment is based on elimination of or reduction in illicit/inappropriate drug use, elimination or marked reduction in illegal activities, improved employment, positive social behavior, and general health. Strikingly lower mortality and morbidity rates are seen in methadone-maintained patients in comparison with untreated addicted populations. Such treatment has been shown to be effective in the reduction of the spread of HIV and other infections from parenteral heroin use. A variant of methadone—

l-alpha-acetylmethadol (LAAM)—has a three-day duration of effect versus methadone's twenty-four hours.

A cadre of doctors today are experts at medication-assisted drug treatments. Their skills include opioid/methadone pharmacology; initial client assessment; dosage induction; stabilization and medically assisted withdrawal; managing poly-substance abuse; methadone take-home dosages; urine drug testing; drug court referrals to methadone maintenance programs; managing medical/psychiatric comorbidity problems among addicts; motivational enhancement for lifestyle changes; and methadone patients living with AIDS and/or HCV infection. High dosages of methadone are proving most effective at reducing heroin use among clients. Methadone maintenance in residential settings is also being applied. New maintenance drugs such as buprenorphine are in the experimental stage. Research is being blended with practice. New federal regulations include provisions to permit expanded medical maintenance treatment for stabilized patients, and program counselors will now have to receive official accreditation. An explicit formulation of principles is long overdue. Methadone maintenance is effective in reducing IDU and needle sharing (Ball et al., 1988). In a report of HIV seropositivity rates among four groups of drug addicts in Bergamo, Italy, patients on methadone maintenance had lower seropositivity rates than those in therapeutic communities, legal custody, or those who were admitted to hospitals for other reasons (Bourne, 1988).

Methadone maintenance programs are more effective in reducing heroin addiction when linked with enriched, comprehensive treatment services. These include professional counseling and well-designed job training and development components (McLellan et al., 1993; Woody et al., 1986; Woody, McLellan, and O'Brien, 1983; Regier and Farmer, 1990).

Unfortunately, these high-quality adjunctive services are not available in many for-profit methadone clinics, which are mainly "filling stations" where clients cruise in, gas up, and "split." To the U.S. Drug Enforcement Administration, methadone is a Class II controlled substance, unavailable for maintenance except in government-licensed and inspected clinics, most of which today are privately owned. Maintenance used to be publicly funded, now it is privatized and conducted out of for-profit operations. Each operation usually owns a string of ten to thirty clinics nationwide, where up to 700 clients on each clinic's caseload pay $200 a month for methadone. Methadone usually is dispensed out of sleazy, low-rent buildings in poor parts of town because neighbors always object to the proximity of these facilities. Profits are good for clinic owners. They have internationalized their operations to Mexican cities such as Tijuana and Ciudad Juárez.

Repeated studies have shown that what is termed "counseling" in many methadone maintenance treatment programs is superficial and does not meet the complex needs of clients (Zweben, 1991). Staff rarely have sufficient diagnostic sophistication, time, or money to identify patients with a need for enhanced services. Many methadone maintenance clients have dual diagnoses of addiction and psychiatric problems. Psychotherapy alone is prohibitively expensive to provide, and rarely controls addiction, but it is better than most of the "counseling" provided. Some clinic owners and staff seem more concerned about money than improving clients' lives. Methadone maintenance program staff are usually poorly trained and low-paid.

The actual cost of a 60 mg daily dose of methadone is 55 cents, or $200 annually. With 700 clients on a clinic caseload each paying over $2,000 a year, the net profit of over $1 million at each clinic after urine testing, rent, paper shuffling, staff salaries, and owner profits could be viewed as excessive. There are over 120,000 addicts on methadone maintenance in New York City alone. Free methadone maintenance would eliminate this money scheme. If it were coupled with aggressive outreach by streetwise ex-addicts, and better services provided by higher qualified staff, clinics would attract more clients who want get "off" heroin.

### 3. Free needle/syringe-exchange programs (NEPs).

Needle scarcity prompts needle sharing, HIV and HCV transmission. NEPs allow drug addicts to swap used needles/syringes for clean ones and should be greatly expanded in America. Today, only about 120 NEPs operate in about seventy-two cities (U.S. Department of Health and Human Services, 1997). Less amounts of needle sharing and lower HIV seroprevalence rates among IDUs and their families have been shown to accompany policies that allow the purchase or free exchange of hypodermic needles without a prescription (Wallace et al., 1998; Hagan and Gormley, 1998; CDC, 1993; Carlson, Siegal, and Falck, 1994; Hagan et al., 1991). A new sterile needle costs about a dime. At the same time, officials of AIDS organizations estimate that the average lifetime cost of treating an individual with HIV/AIDS is at least $119,000. A significant preponderance of recent evidence (Lurie, Drucker, and Knowles, 1998; Vlahov et al., 1998; Selwyn, 1988) further strengthens the effectiveness of NEPs and the paucity of associated adverse effects. *No measurable increase in intravenous heroin use follows implementation of NEPs; they do not encourage drug use.* Researchers at the Albert Einstein College of Medicine in New York estimate that as many as 10,000 HIV infections could have been prevented between 1987 and 1995 had programs that supply clean needles to addicts been generally available (Bennett, 1995).

Such an estimate of lives saved through NEPs assuredly *underestimates* the potential effectiveness of syringe exchanges. The National Institutes of Health reports that existing NEPs have brought about an estimated 30 percent or greater reduction of HIV infection in IDUs. Not only could lives be saved, but hundreds of millions of dollars in AIDS treatment costs would be saved by preventing new HIV infections through the clean-needle approach.

At present, needle distribution without prescription is illegal in at least nine states, and nearly all states have laws prohibiting carrying drug paraphernalia. There currently is a ban on federal funding of NEPs. In the penumbra of these successes, the U.S. Conference of Mayors has urged elimination of the ban on federal funding for NEPs. Needle-exchange programs alone will not stop IDU, but they help in reducing the spread of HIV—and that needs to be a priority. In California, Governor Gray Davis and ex-Attorney General Dan Lungren (with undisguised venom) have aggressively opposed NEPs, but local officials in San Francisco and Oakland support and allow them. Nationwide, the number of NEPs continues to grow slowly, some operate either illegally or on the fringe of the law. The combination of NEPs, efforts to increase syringe availability by modifying restrictive laws and regulations, and outreach to increase pharmacist involvement in syringe sales continues to hold promise for reducing the toll of HIV and HCV infection among IDUs, their sex partners, and their children.

## 4. Decriminalize heroin.

Heroin decriminalization is a public policy option worth consideration. For example, addicts could come in to a clinic, be supplied with maintenance doses of heroin, and then some of them could be transferred to oral methadone. The logic of decriminalization depends on two assumptions: 1) that heroin is not as dangerous to the user as it is popularly believed, and 2) that the drug and risky methods of consumption are unlikely to prove appealing to many people, precisely because they are so obviously dangerous.

Since the 1920s, the so-called "heroin problem" has sprung from class and culture conflict over the distribution of opportunities in society and over approved forms of recreation and entertainment. Heroin is a relatively safe drug, compared with alcohol and tobacco. Addicts can lead productive lives. Take the case of William Stewart Halsted, a doyen of American surgery and founder and chairman of the Surgery Department at Johns Hopkins University. Famous and respected as the inventor of rubber surgical gloves, the use of silk sutures, the radical operation for breast cancer, a prototype operation for inguinal hernia, and numerous other important surgical contributions, Halsted was riven by heavy *legal* morphine addiction well into his eighties (Wangensteen and Wangensteen, 1978; Olch, 1975; Ravitch, 1986).

Many assert that the criminalization of heroin causes more harm than the drug itself, including: ex-federal prosecutor and former mayor of Baltimore Kurt Schmoke, Milton Friedman, William F. Buckley, former U.S. Secretary of State George Schultz, former U.N. Secretary-General Javier Perez de Cuellar, New Mexico Governor Gary Johnson, former FDA Commissioner and Stanford President Donald Kennedy, Walter Cronkite, the Reverend George Schiller— and many more (Nadelmann, 1988). Critics call heroin illegalization an aspect of American puritanism, and point to the enormous increase in the number of prisoners serving sentences for drug-related crimes—an elevenfold jump between 1980 and 1996 (Texeira, 2000), with African Americans bearing the brunt.

The argument for heroin decriminalization is not new. General Barry McCaffrey, much-decorated soldier and President Clinton's ex-drug czar, embodied the case against decriminalization.

Do you mean that you support having industrial-quality meth-amphetamines available at a 7-Eleven in your community for your 18-year-old son or employee? It's an elitist argument to say drug abuse doesn't affect me and my kind, that if you just legalize it, the problem will go away. (Winik, 2000, p. 6)

Such pronouncements remind one of the Bible-thumping preacher whose notes read: "argument here weak; shout like hell." McCaffrey's proposed replacement, John P. Walters, who served as a deputy to two antidrug czars in the first Bush administration, has also championed hawkish antidrug measures in the nation's $20 billion drug law enforcement war. In response to the statistic of African Americans being thirteen times more likely to be imprisoned for drug offenses than whites, he dismissed this as an urban myth (Wisnia, 2001). In addition, Walters proposes pulling licenses of doctors prescribing medical marijuana, and calls treating addicts "the latest manifestation of the liberals' commitment to a therapeutic state" ("A Little Drug War Quiz," 2001).

The dicta of the generals and drug fighters notwithstanding, dogmas which are light on substance but long on self-promotion, derail any attempts at decreasing narcotic use and addiction. The conclusion that decriminalization will extend the use of narcotics has been inaccurate for some time. The argument that availability will parallel increase of addiction is not consonant with the data from other countries; the Netherlands and Switzerland, for example.

The case for decriminalization, however, is endorsed by many respected politicians, law-enforcement officials, public health experts, and scholars on both sides of the political aisle. They note that as with the previous liquor prohibition, the destructive result of illegal heroin markets is corruption. Counternarcotics forces, such as those in Mexico, "trade" enforcement for a share of the take.

Legal heroin maintenance would slash crime, misery, and death associated with the heroin scene. In 1999, the legal dispensing of heroin to addicts in Switzerland led to improvements in health among them and reductions in addiction-related crime. The death toll from overdose and IDU-associated diseases among an estimated 30,000 Swiss heroin addicts has also dropped (Bruellman, 1999). However, no control group was used to determine whether the heroin prescription was a factor in crime reduction and health improvements.

Voters in Switzerland in 1997 overwhelmingly endorsed the government's liberal heroin maintenance policies. The Swiss placed their heroin program on a permanent legal footing in 1998, four years after the first experimental distributions. Swiss addicts are given prescribed doses of heroin. Their program proves that it is medically feasible to prescribe intravenous heroin as a maintenance drug.

Heroin maintenance is not capitulation to the drug traffickers. On the contrary, it is just the opposite. It would reduce the illegal heroin business, and concomitant profits would slide. In the cold spotlight of the clear results in other developed countries, the advantages of the decriminalization strategy far outweigh those of current and planned U.S. policies. There is abundant evidence that decriminalization of the drug is the optimal way to attack the heroin problem, if this is indeed the intention of the "war on drugs" (Nadelmann, 1988).

If heroin were available to designated addicts in pharmacies, even liquor stores, or as an over-the-counter drug (Kaplan, 1983; Trebach, 1982), the present incentive which underlies the narcotics industry would be curtailed. Repealing antiheroin laws as they apply to bona fide addicts will *not* lead to a big rise in drug abuse. There is no evidence that "clean" Americans would inject heroin even if it were legal.

Decriminalizing heroin would require an almost unimaginable sea change of sociopolitical reform. Heroin maintenance would have to be acceptable to real policymakers in the real world. The rational model of policy analysis depends on the ability of public decision makers to respond to rational arguments, to adopt strategies that achieve a given social goal in the most effective and efficient manner. The audience for heroin decriminalization consists of real-world government officials, who are subject to the forces of popular opinion and interest groups. The public has exerted enormous pressure on these officials that seems to preclude any independent exercise of judgment on the heroin question. Recommendations are not rational abstractions addressed to hypothetical policymakers who operate without political constraints. Rather, they are directed to real decision makers, in the real political environment, and heroin decriminalization is not a realistic option in the present political context. It would be political suicide for a public official to endorse it. People still seem to want heroin to remain illegal. Do they really want prison cells to be filled by sickly old men, who are unlikely to commit any further crimes, and with minor heroin dealers who will inevitably be replaced by other dealers after their arrest?

## 5. Reform prostitution laws.

Reform of punitive antiprostitution laws would prevent HIV/AIDS and HCV infection, provide better child care, reproductive health care, and eventuate in less illicit drug abuse among FSWs. This goes right along with heroin decriminalization.

No official definition of legalized or (decriminalized) prostitution exists. "Legalization" means any alternative to absolute criminalization. This could range from the licensing of brothels and street prostitution to the absence of *any* laws against prostitution. Most references to law reform in the media and in other contemporary contexts use the term "legalization" to refer to a system of criminal regulation and government control of prostitutes, wherein certain prostitutes are given licenses which permit them to work in specific and usually limited ways. "Decriminalization" usually means the removal of laws against prostitution. It is often used to refer to total decriminalization, that is, the repeal of laws against consensual adult sexual activity, in commercial and noncommercial contexts. Advocates for the new prostitutes' rights movement call for decriminalization of all aspects of prostitution resulting from individual decisions. "Legalization" often includes special taxes for prostitutes, restricting prostitutes to working in brothels or in certain zones, licenses, registration of prostitutes (and fees for such registration), government records of individual prostitutes, and periodic health examinations for STDs. In Mexico, legalization means that prostitution is not against the law.

According to reformers, FSWs should pay income and business taxes, form unions, earn Social Security and medical benefits. They should have access to counseling relative to job change and to training for other occupations. Outside the United States every one of these reforms has been tried, tested, and found to be eminently workable and productive.

Legalized prostitution is not a foreseeable option in this era, however. The Puritan strain runs deep in American culture, and its legacy is evident in the criminalization of prostitution, as with other early taboos against dancing, card playing, and drinking. For the United States's Puritan founders—as nineteenth-century French historian

Alexis de Tocqueville observed, the chief care was the maintenance of orderly conduct and good morals in the community.

FSWs currently suffer from occupational safety and health hazards that include:

- Personal injuries such as repetitive stress injuries from performing fellatio and "hand jobs."
- Bladder/kidney infections from repeated traumatic vaginal intercourse.
- Foot and back problems from street FSWs' prolonged standing and walking on high heels.
- Job-related emotional stress from working in an illegal market without paid sick leaves, workers' compensation or disability insurance, paid vacation, or minimum wage, and concomitant fear of arrest.
- Drug and alcohol dependency related to client demand and/or job stress. (Alexander, Highleyman, and La Croix, 1996)

Five hundred thousand female prostitutes work in Germany, which has a population of 82 million (Williams, 1999). One in 160 German women is a prostitute. Germany is at the forefront in its liberal approach to commercial sex work. Prostitutes will soon qualify there for state health insurance, pensions, and Social Security. Brothels are legitimate, taxpaying businesses. Other changes being considered would eliminate prostitution-free zones.

FSWs in the Netherlands already enjoy most of these social protections, but few other European countries have taken up the banner of social justice for this segment of the population, long relegated to the fringes. In fact, in 1999, liberal Sweden recriminalized prostitution after a long-standing policy of tolerance and made those soliciting sex for money liable for hefty fines. Many from the political right are opposed to equal rights and social insurance for prostitutes on economic as well as moral grounds.

All sex workers, male and female, should be required to have periodic health screenings for sexually transmitted diseases. However, laws excluding HIV positive people from working as prostitutes may be counterproductive in HIV prevention work. Such measures can encourage prostitutes to go underground if they think they may be

HIV positive. HIV positive prostitutes still have to work. They have to be carefully counseled to use condoms.

A low HIV seropositivity rate exists in female prostitutes who do not inject drugs, as evidenced by the studies in Mexico. The assumption is often made that prostitutes are at greater risk of HIV infection because of their multiple sex partners. It is also assumed that prostitutes spread HIV to their clients and thus play a major role in transmitting the virus into the heterosexual population. This is true to a certain extent, but studies of a number of countries have shown that FSWs who are not IDUs do not have a high prevalence of HIV, and in nations where prostitution is decriminalized most prostitutes report high levels of condom use with their clients.

Prostitutes' rights advocates argue that all aspects of adult prostitution resulting from individual decisions should be decriminalized, and third parties should be regulated according to standard business codes. Existing business codes allow abuse of sex workers. Criminal laws against fraud and coercion should be enforced. In places where soliciting is a criminal offense, it reduces the time prostitutes have for negotiation with their clients. This puts them at risk for criminal attack by some johns. Intensive policing has led to prostitution in more remote areas where they are even more vulnerable to attack, and excluded from HIV prevention/education workers.

In terms of working conditions, decriminalization advocates say that review of sex work as legitimate employment is long overdue. It is only beginning to be reconsidered in the context of the historically limited employment opportunities for women. Why can't prostitution be a legitimate job and brothels valid workplaces (Albert, 2000)? Nevada's legal brothels, for example, are clean, legitimate workplaces where the women are not shackled hostages (except in terms of obedience to workplace rules, like everybody else), but self-aware professionals there of their own free will. The troubles they face at work—from long hours away from their families to lack of health benefits and overtime compensation—are just like the problems many low-skilled American workers experience on the job. Prostitutes should have unemployment insurance, health insurance, and housing. Laws and ordinances which imply systematically zoning out prostitution should be carefully reconsidered and redrawn to establish zones of toleration. (Phederson, 1989). Laws discriminating against prostitutes associating and working collectively in order to acquire a higher degree of personal security should be abolished. Organizations of prostitutes and ex-prostitutes should be supported to further implement reforms.

Employment counseling, legal, and housing services for runaway children should be funded to prevent child prostitution and to promote child well-being and opportunity. Shelters and services for working prostitutes and retraining programs for prostitutes who want to leave "the life" should be funded and available.

No special taxes should be levied on prostitutes, but legal brothels may be subject to such levies, as they are in Nevada. Prostitutes should pay regular taxes on the same basis as other independent contractors and employees, and should receive the same benefits, such as Social Security, Medicaid, and at retirement, Medicare.

Educational programs to change social attitudes which stigmatize and discriminate against sex workers and ex-sex workers should be supported. Such programs would help the public to understand that the customer plays a crucial role in the prostitution phenomenon. This role, at present, is generally ignored. The customer, like the prostitute, should not, however, be criminalized or condemned on a moral basis. The arrest of "johns," publication of their names in newspapers, seizure of their automobiles, and other punitive actions against them should be stopped.

At this moment, FSWs are trying to address their needs in the areas of basic necessities, legal support, and psychological counseling. A frank appraisal indicates that FSWs want to improve self-esteem, self-determination, and greater access to civil rights through action aimed at combating stigma and violence against them. Few governments have addressed the central issue of sex workers' control over their work.

What about popular support? Some opinion surveys show that the public favors prostitution decriminalization. In a San Francisco telephone poll of over 10,000 calls, 85 percent supported legalization of prostitution ("85 Percent Support," 1993). U.S. policymakers would do well to emulate the sex worker health licensing model in the Mexican cities where interviews were conducted for this book. There is an urgent need for an integrated, risk-reduction program among American FSWs focusing on regular HIV/STD checkups, safe-sex practices, and drug abuse prevention, treatment, and rehabilitation programs targeting this high-risk population.

## CONCLUSIONS

Heroin maintenance, NEPs, and prostitution law reforms have conflicted with highly visible and dramatically publicized increases in drug and prostitution enforcement over the past few years, which have had little effect. In fact, drug and prostitution enforcement have backfired. They promote riskier behavior.

Drug and prostitution control policies are highly costly and counterproductive. Current efforts to reduce these ancient behaviors must be abandoned, the slate wiped clean, and other approaches adopted.

Eliminating drug crops and trafficking routes, and interdicting street prostitutes, is an exercise in futility. Restricting FSWs and drug supplies only shifts operations to other locations to meet the demand (and to technologies such as cell phones and pagers). The process cannot be stopped—not with all the lawyers, "drug czars," guns, and money in the world. Not with crime summits, or blue-ribbon task forces, or committees. Not with bullets, preachings of morality, or by righteous indignation. The heroin and sex businesses will burgeon at the same old stand in the same old way.

### The "Drug Abuse Industrial Complex": Complicit Partners in Wrongdoing

The money spent by the United States on chasing, prosecuting, incarcerating, and treating heroin addicts and FSWs is substantial. The federal government spends over $20 billion a year on drug control, but only $6.1 billion of it (33.4 percent) for "demand reduction" prevention, treatment, and rehabilitation programs. These supply reduction costs are in addition to city, county, and state-funded supply reduction programs. When added to city, county, and state costs of capturing, arresting, trying, convicting, and incarcerating heroin distributors, users, and abusers, together with the aggregate dollar outlay for controlling heroin supply and demand, the total financial drug-fighting cost becomes enormous. "Fighting heroin" creates over-world (and *underworld*) economic pressure groups who develop vital interests in *sustaining* the addiction "problem" and vitiate attempts at policy reform such as heroin decriminalization, which may be the most rational approach.

The benighted relationship of business to "defense" was highlighted by President Dwight Eisenhower on January 17, 1961, in his farewell radio and television address when he coined the term "military-industrial complex":

> In the councils of government, we must guard against the acquisition of unwarranted influence, whether sought or unsought, by the military-industrial complex. The potential for the disastrous rise of misplaced power exists and will persist. (Eisenhower, 1961, p. 216)

Eisenhower could not at that time allude to a similar titanic complex in the social services field. "The education-poverty-mental health industrial complex" (Shapiro, 1975; Stockman, 1975) is a social pork barrel consisting of a broad array of groups whose basic industry is ministering to the psychosocial problems of poverty. This social pork barrel, argued Shapiro, "just like the military-industrial complex, makes thousands of workers dependent on the federal budget for their jobs and way of life" (Shapiro, 1975, p. 25).

In 1973, the term "drug abuse industrial complex" was coined, and referred to the combined economic effect of federal drug law enforcement and addiction treatment efforts (Sonnenreich, 1973). Fighting prostitution, with its close association to substance abuse, is part of this industry.

The "turnkey industry" of busting addicts and prostitutes is a profitable enterprise for customs agents, police, court personnel, correctional institutions, attorneys, and peripheral hangers-on: bail bondsmen, jail and prison construction contractors, prison guards and their politically powerful unions, urine-testing labs, and even some ex-offender programs. It provides thousands of jobs for middle-class Americans. Politicians manipulate drug and prostitution issues to win votes. Private security firms, burglar alarm companies, theft detection/prevention manufacturers, and insurance companies tap deeply held public fears and end up turning handsome profits.

Though the stated goal of this turnkey industry is to self-destruct, its unstated mission is self-perpetuation. Quite simply, the criminal justice system needs addicts and prostitutes and has developed what is called a "vested interest" in maintaining addiction and the sex industry. If addiction and commercial sex disappeared tomorrow, many police officers and their ancillary personnel would be out of jobs.

The north American prostitute lurches from one compelling pressure to another. She lives between the physical need for illicit drugs and her vulnerability to STDs. She cowers under the authority of police, but must shut up and take it.

In Mexico the FSW has a relatively better deal. She conducts her trade fairly openly, albeit in her agreed-upon business area. She is not segregated as a pariah. Her profession is as open to scrutiny as a doctor or grocer. She is not maligned as immoral or miscreant, because the culture in which she lives recognizes the ineffectiveness of prohibiting her services, which are as old as humanity. The fact is she does not have to run and hide, and a need for drugs is not a thread in her tapestry.

The expected result of all this is less AIDS and other STDs among the Mexican FSWs than among similar tradespeople in the United States. A lonesome marine on leave is less likely to be infected in Tijuana than in San Bernardino, California.

The most salient difference in the way that prostitution is viewed between the two countries is the splenetic intolerance in the United States. This viewpoint, as has been demonstrated, perpetuates dissemination of STDs.

This book is not a brief in favor of prostitution in as much as it recognizes its need for existence and for toleration. The more open-minded Mexican public policies on commercial sex work should be emulated by U.S. legislators. To reduce AIDS, hepatitis C, and other STDs among American FSWs, a Mexican-style commercial sex work decriminalization and registration system should be considered. Expanded needle exchange and free methadone and heroin maintenance are also recommended. However, political, economic, and moral constraints color the context of these decisions, making them unlikely in the near future.

For now, the United States is stuck in neutral. To be searingly candid, mind-altering drugs and sex for sale are here to stay. When our legislators, on their high road of rectitude and probity, responding to the puritanical ethos of the citizenry recognize this and employ the Mexican blueprint, a significant dent will be made in the spread of disease.

# Appendix

# Survey Questionnaire

I. BACKGROUND CHARACTERISTICS/CRIMINAL HISTORY
   1. Age: _____
   2. Education: _____
   3. Married: _____
   4. Boyfriend: _____
   5. Race/ethnic group:
      (a) Anglo: _____
      (b) Black: _____
      (c) Hispanic: _____
      (d) Asian: _____
   6. Duration of prostitution: _____
   7. Number of arrests: _____
   8. Number of convictions: _____
   9. Done time: _____

II. DRUG USE HISTORY
   10. Have you ever used IV drugs: _____
   11. Are you using IV drugs now: _____ (if no, skip to #17)
   12. What drugs do you inject:
      (a) heroin: _____
      (b) cocaine: _____
      (c) meth: _____
      (d) barbs _____
      (e) none _____
   13. Husband/boyfriend(s) IDU:
      (a) No husband/boyfriend(s) _____ (if no, skip to #15)
      (b) If husband/boyfriend(s), use IV drugs? _____
   14. Do you share an outfit with them: _____
   15. Do you share an outfit with any other people: _____
      (a) If yes, how many people: _____
   16. Would you like to clean up: _____

III.  BRIEF MEDICAL HISTORY
    17. Number of children:____
    18. Medical checks:
        (a)  weekly:____
        (b)  every two weeks:____
        (c)  every three weeks:____
        (d)  monthly: ____
        (e)  now and then: ____
        (f)  never: ____
    19. Ever had a positive test for syphilis:____
    20. Ever had gonorrhea:____
    21. Ever had herpes: ____
    22. Have you ever heard of AIDS: ____
    23. How can you get AIDS: ____
        (a)  unprotected sex:____
        (b)  injecting drugs:____
        (c)  sex and drugs: ____
        (d)  don't know: ____
    24. Have you ever had a blood test for AIDS: ____
        (a)  If yes, longer than a month ago: ____
        b)  If yes, positive or negative: ____
    25. If you have not been tested for AIDS, would you like to be tested
        for it:
        (a)  very much:____
        (b)  not much: ____
        (c)  not at all:____
    26. Have you heard of anybody in the prostitute community around
        here getting AIDS over the last five years or so:____
    27. Have you heard of anybody in the prostitute community around
        here dying of AIDS in the last five years or so:____
IV. SEXUAL BEHAVIOR WITH CUSTOMERS
    28. What do you do with most of your customers:
        (a)  penis-vaginal intercourse:____
        (b)  penis-oral intercourse: ____
        (c)  penis-rectal intercourse: ____
        (d)  oral-vaginal kissing: ____
        (e)  hand job:____
        (f)  other: ____

29. How many customers per day on the average:____
30. Average charge for service: $____
31. Amount of habit (if applicable):$____
32. Do you take any precautions with customers so you don't catch a sexually transmitted disease:
    (a) request customers wear condom:_____
    (b) require customers wear condom:_____
    (c) inspect customers for signs of venereal disease:____
    (d) none: ____
    (e) other:____
33. How do most of your customers feel about wearing condoms:
    (a) most don't like to wear them:____
    (b) more want to use them lately:____
    (c) most want to use them: ____
    (d) don't know: ____
34. How many of your customers originally insist on intercourse without condoms:____
35. Has there been any change in the last year or so in the number of customers who bring up the subject of AIDS:
    (a) no change:____
    (b) more bring it up:____
36. What percent of your new customers bring up the subject of AIDS:____
37. What percent of new customers ask you if you've been tested for AIDS:____
38. What percent of your customers do you think are afraid of catching AIDS from a prostitute:____
39. What are most of your customers:
    (a) businessmen: ____
    (b) professionals:____
    (c) blue collar: ____
40. Are most of your customers:
    (a) Anglo:____
    (b) Black:____
    (c) Hispanic:____
    (d) Asian:____
    (e) Native Am:____
V. FEAR OF AIDS
41. Are you afraid at all of catching AIDS:
    (a) very much:____
    (b) some:____
    (c) not at all:____

42. Are any other prostitutes and/or IV drug users you know afraid of catching AIDS:_____
43. Has anyone you know stopped shooting drugs or prostituting because they are afraid of catching AIDS:___
44. If you got AIDS, how do you think you would have gotten it:
    (a) sex:_____
    (b) sex and shooting drugs:_____
    (c) shooting drugs:_____
    (d) don't know: _____
45. If you wanted to make sure you never caught AIDS, what do you think you should do:
    (a) stop hooking:_____
    (b) stop shooting drugs:_____
    (c) stop hooking and shooting drugs:_____
    (d) don't share outfit:_____
    (e) other: _____
    (f) don't know:___
46. If you had AIDS, would you keep working the street?_____
47. Is there anything you think should be done so people like you would have less chance of catching AIDS?

    _____

48. SUMMARY NOTES:

    _____

# References

"85 Percent Support Legalization of Prostitution." 1993. *San Francisco Examiner,* December 7, p. A1.

"A Little Drug War Quiz." Editorial. 2001. *Los Angeles Times,* September 11, p. B8.

Albert, Alexa E. 2000. *BROTHEL: Mustang Ranch and Its Women.* New York: Random House.

Albert, Alexa E., David Lee Warner, Robert A. Hatcher, James Trussell, and Charles Bennett. 1995. "Condom Use Among Female Commercial Sex Workers in Nevada's Legal Brothels." Unpublished paper. Family Planning Program, Emory University School of Medicine.

Alexander, Priscilla, Liz Highleyman, and Catherine La Croix. 1996. "Occupational Safety and Health Regulations As an HIV/AIDS Prevention Strategy in the Context of Sex Work." *XI International Conference on AIDS, Abstracts-on-Disk.* Whitehouse Station, NJ: Merck and Co.

Alter, Miriam J. 1995. Epidemiology of Hepatitis C in the West. *Seminar on Liver Disease,* 15 (January 4): 5-14.

Alter, Miriam J. 1997. "Hepatitis C: The Clinical Spectrum of Disease." National Institutes of Health Conference on Hepatitis C, Bethesda, Maryland.

American Health Consultants, 2001. *Emergency Medicine Reports,* 22 (no. 12), June 4, p. 1.

Anslinger, Harry J. and William F. Tomkins. 1953. *The Traffic in Narcotics.* New York: Funk and Wagnalls.

Badillo, Armando Ruíz, C. Magis-Rodriguez, R. Ortiz Mondragon, R. Lozada-Romero, P. E. Uribe Zuniga. 1998. "Persons Who Inject Drugs in Treatment and Prisoners in Tijuana, Baja California, Mexico." *12th World AIDS Conference, Abstracts-on-Disk.* Whitehouse Station, NJ: Merck and Co.

Ball, John C., D. P. Francis, H. W. Jaffe, P. N. Fultz, J. P. Getchell, J. S. McDougal, and P. M. Feorino. 1988. Reducing the Risk of AIDS Through Methadone Maintenance Treatment. *Journal of Health and Social Behavior,* 29(1): 214-226.

Bellis, David J. 1983. *Heroin and Politicians: The Failure of Public Policy to Control Addiction in America.* Westport, CT: Greenwood Press.

_____. 1989. The Impact of AIDS Fear on Behavior Change Among Heroin-Addicted Female Prostitutes: Street Interviews With 72 Subjects, *Journal of the Western Governmental Research Association,* 5 (Spring): 4-36.

_____. 1990. Fear of AIDS and Risk Reduction Among Heroin-Addicted Female Street Prostitutes: Personal Interviews with 72 Southern California Subjects. *Journal of Alcohol and Drug Education,* 35(3): 26-37.

_____. 1993. Reduction of AIDS Risk Among 41 Heroin-Addicted Female Street Prostitutes: Effects of Free Methadone Maintenance, *Journal of Addictive Diseases,* 12(1): 26-37.

_____. 2001. HIV/AIDS Risk Behavior of Female Sex Workers in Mexico: Comparison of Interviews with a Cohort Study in San Bernardino, Califorina. *Journal of Borderlands Studies,* 16 (no. 1): 83-96.

Benjamin, Harry and R. E. L. Masters. 1964. *Prostitution and Morality: A Definitive Report on the Prostitute in Contemporary Society and an Analysis of the Causes and Effects of the Suppression of Prostitution.* New York: The Julian Press.

Bennett, Amanda. 1995. "Needle-Swap Programs Spark Life-and-Death Debates." *The Wall Street Journal.* July 10, p. B1.

Bertram, Eva and Kenneth Sharpe. 1998. "The Drug War Corrupts Absolutely." *Los Angeles Times,* October 4, p. M2.

_____. 1999. "Escalation = More Drugs." *The Nation,* March 29, pp. 6-7.

Booth, Robert E., Thomas J. Crowley, and Yiming Zhang. 1996. Substance Abuse Treatment Entry, Retention and Effectiveness: Out-of-Treatment Opiate Injection Drug Users. *Drug and Alcohol Dependence,* 42(1): 11-20.

Booth, William. 1988a. AIDS and Drug Abuse: No Quick Fix. *Science,* 239(2): 717-719.

_____. 1988b. CDC Painting a Picture of HIV Infection in the United States. *Science,* 239(1): 253.

Bourne, Peter G. 1988. AIDS and Drug Use: An International Perspective. *Journal of Psychoactive Drugs,* 20(2): 153-157.

Bruellman, Matthias. 1999. "Switzerland Still Cautious About Success Of Heroin Program." *San Bernardino County Sun,* April 17, p. A4.

Bullough, Vern L. 1964. *The History of Prostitution.* New York: University Books.

Burroughs, William S. 1959. *Naked Lunch.* New York: Grove Press.

Caldwell, John C. and Pat Caldwell. 1996. The African AIDS Epidemic. *Scientific American,* 274(3): 62-68.

Carlson, Robert G., Harvey A. Siegal, and Russell S. Falck. 1994. Ethnography, Epidemiology, and Public Policy: Needle-Use Practices and HIV-1 Risk Reduction Among Injecting Drug Users in the Midwest. In Douglas A. Feldman (Ed.), *Global AIDS Policy,* pp. 185-214. Westport, CT: Bergin and Garvey.

Centers for Disease Control and Prevention. 1985. Heterosexual Transmission of Human T-Lymphotropic Virus Type III/Lymphadenopathy-Associated Virus. *MMWR,* 34(37): 561-563.

_____. 1986. Update: Acquired Immunodeficiency Syndrome—United States. *MMWR,* 36(49): 757-766.

_____. 1987a. Antibody to Human Immunodeficiency Virus in Female Prostitutes. *MMWR,* 36(11): 801-804.

_____. 1987b. Human Immunodeficiency Virus Infection in Transfusion Recipients and Their Family members. *MMWR,* 36(10): 137-140.

_____. 1987c. Human Immunodeficiency Virus in the United States. *MMWR,* 36(49): 801-804.

_____. 1988. Recommendations for Prevention and Control of Hepatitis C Virus (HCV) Infection and HCV-Related Chronic Disease. *Morbidity and Mortality Weekly Report (MMWR),* 37(RR-19): 1-39.

_____. 1993. "The Public Health Impact of Needle Exchange Programs in the United States and Abroad," 1 and 2. Washington, DC: U.S. Department of Health and Human Services.

_____. 1995. *HIV/AIDS Surveillance Report,* 7 (2): 1-39.

_____. 2001. Press Release: "20 Years of AIDS: 450,000 Americans Dead, over 1 million have been infected." Author.

Cimons, Marlene. 1998. "AIDS Falls Off List of Top 10 Killers in U.S." *Los Angeles Times,* October 8, p. 1A.

_____. 1999. "FDA Approves First Home Kit to Test for Hepatitis C." *Los Angeles Times,* April 30, p. A10.

_____. 2001. "Data on AIDS May Suggest Resurgence." *Los Angeles Times,* June 1, p. A22.

City and County of San Francisco. 1996. San Francisco Task Force on Prostitution. *Final Report 1996: Summary of Recommendations.* San Francisco: City and County of San Francisco.

Clumeck, Nathan, Marjorie Robert-Gurnoff, Philippe Van De Perre, Andrea Jennings, Jean Sibomana, Patrick Demol, Sophie Cran, and Robert C. Gallo. 1985. Seroepidemiological Studies Among Selected Groups of Heterosexual Africans. *Journal of the American Medical Association,* 254 (November 8): 2600-2601.

Cockburn, Alexander and Jeffrey St. Clair. 1998. *The CIA, Drugs, and the Press.* New York: Verso Press.

Colón, Hector, Hardeo Sahai, Rafaela R. Robles, and Tomás D. Matos. 1995. Effects of a Community Outreach Program in HIV Risk Behaviors Among Injection Drug Users in San Juan, Puerto Rico: An analysis of Trends. *AIDS Education and Prevention,* 7(3): 195-209.

Connell, Rich and Robert J. Lopez. 1996. "Gang Finds Safe Haven and Base for Operations in Tijuana." *Los Angeles Times.* November 19, p. A18.

Cowan, Martin J., Anthony Divittis, Lee Kochems, Peter Mastrionni, Kevin Mahony, and Charles McKinney. 1984. Maternal Transmission of Acquired Immunodeficiency Syndrome. *Pediatrics,* 73 (March 3): 382-386.

Craig, Richard. 1989. U.S. Narcotics Policy Toward Mexico: Consequences for the Bilateral Relationship. In Guadalup Gonzalez and Marta Tienda (Eds.), *The Drug Connection in U.S.-Mexican Relations.* San Diego: Bilaterial Commission on the Future of United States-Mexican Relations, UCSD.

"Crisis y Demografia." 1998. *Excelsiór, El Periódico de la Vida Nacionál.* May 11, p. 1-F.

Cruz-Valdez, Aurelio, M. Castaneda, V. Tovar-Guzman, L. Rivera-Rivera, M. Quiterio-Trenado, and B. Allen. 1998. "Knowledge of HIV transmission and prevention among Mexican adolescents." *12th World AIDS Conference, Abstracts-on-Disk.* Whitehouse Station, NJ: Merck and Co.

Curran, James W., Harold W. Jaffe, Ann M. Hardy, W. Meade Morgan, Richard M. Selik, and Timothy J. Dondero. 1988. Epidemiology of HIV Infection and AIDS in the United States. *Science,* 239(2): 610-616.

Dahlberg, John-Thor and Mary Beth Sheridan. 1998. "Swiss Allege Raul Salinas Is a Drug Kingpin." *Los Angeles Times,* October 21, p. A1.

De Córdoba, José and Margaret Studer, 1998. "Swiss Link Raul Salinas to Drugs, Confiscate $114.4 Million in Assets." *The Wall Street Journal,* October 21, p. A17.

Dean-Gaitor, Hazel, P.L.F. Fleming, and J.W.W. Ward. 1998. "Trends in AIDS Incidence Among Black Persons - United States, 1990-1996." *12th World AIDS Conference, Abstracts-on-Disk.* Whitehouse Station, NJ: Merck and Co.

Decker, John F. 1979. *Prostitution: Regulation and Control.* Littleton, CO: Fred B. Rothman.

De Jarlais, Don C., and Samuel R. Friedman. 1988. The Psychology of Preventing AIDS Among Intravenous Drug Users: A Social Learning Conceptualization. *American Psychologist,* 43(11): 865-870.

Delgado, José. 1969. *Physical Control of the Mind: Toward a Psychocivilized Society.* New York: Harper and Row.

Del Rio-Zolezzi, Aurora. 1995. La Epidemia de VIH/SIDA Y La Mujer en México. *Jornál de Salúd Pública de México,* 37: 581-591.

Denis, Francois, Guy Gershy-Damet, Michel Lhuillier, Guy Leonard, Alain Goudeau, Max Essex, Rancis Barin, Jean-Loup Rey, Marcelle Mounier, Affoue Sangare, et al. 1987. Prevalence of Human T-Lymphotropic Retroviruses Type III (HIV) and Type IV in Ivory Coast. *The Lancet* II (February 21): 409.

Deren, Sherry, Michele Shedlin, W. Rees Davis, Michael C. Clatts, Salvador Balcorta, Mark M. Beardsley, Jesus Sanchez, and Don Des Jarlais. 1997. Dominican, Mexican, and Puerto Rican Prostitutes: Drug Use and Sexual Behaviors. *Hispanic Journal of Behavioral Sciences,* 19(2, May): 202-213.

Dicks, Barbara A. 1994. African American Women and AIDS: A Public Health/Social Work Challenge. *Social Work in Health Care,* 19 (3/4): 123-143.

Dirección Generál de Epidemiologia y Instituto Mexicano de Psiquiatria. 1989. *Encuestra Nacionál de Adicciones.* 3 vols. México, DF: Secretaría de Salúd Pública.

Dirección Generál de Epidemiologia/CONASIDA. 1996. *Situación Epidemiologica del SIDA,* 1(3). Mexico, DF: Dirección Generál de Epidemiologia/ CONASIDA.

Dole, Vincent P. 1966. Rehabilitation of Heroin Addicts After Blockade with Methadone. *New York State Journal of Medicine,* 66(April): 2011-2017.

_____. 1967. Heroin Addiction: A Metabolic Disease. *Archives of Internal Medicine,* 120(July): 19-24.

_____. 1976. Methadone Maintenance Treatment: A Ten-Year Perspective. *Journal of the American Medical Association,* 235(May 10): 2117.

_____. 1997. What Is 'Methadone Maintenance Treatment'? *Journal of Maintenance in the Addictions,* 1(1): 7-8.

Dole, Vincent P. and Marie E. Nyswander. 1965. A medical Treatment for Diacetyl Morphine ('Heroin') Addiction. *Journal of the American Medical Association,* 193(August 23): 646-650.

"Don't Let Up in War on AIDS." 1998. *Los Angeles Times.* Editorial. February 4, p. B-6

Duster, Troy. 1970. *The Legislation of Morality: Law, Drugs, and Moral Judgment.* New York: The Free Press.

Dye, Thomas R. 1992. *Understanding Public Policy.* Englewood Cliffs, NY: Prentice-Hall.

Eisenhower, Dwight D. 1961. *Public Papers of the Presidents of the United States, Dwight D. Eisenhower, 1960-1961.* Washington, DC: U.S. Government Printing Office.

Ellingwood, Ken. 1999. "Baja Office Resigns Under Fire." *Los Angeles Times,* July 15, p. A3.

_____. 2000a. "Agency to Address Border Health Issues." *Los Angeles Times,* February 2, p. A35.

_____. 2000b. "Agents' Deaths Underscore Peril of Mexican Drug War." *Los Angeles Times,* May 2, p. A1.

_____. 2000c. "Tijuana Arrestee Said to Be a Founder of Drug Cartel." *Los Angeles Times,* March 16, p. A16.

_____. 2000d. "Tijuana Mourns Its Slain Police Chief." *Los Angeles Times,* March 1, p. A3.

Ellingwood, Ken and Erick Lightblau. 1998. "18 Slain Execution-Style at Farm Near Ensenada." *Los Angeles Times,* September 18, p. A1.

Ellingwood, Ken and Tony Perry. 2000. "Tijuana Police Chief Slain in Hail of Gunfire." *Los Angeles Times,* February 28, p. A1.

"El problema fundamentál de la nación es el crimen organizado."1998. *La Jornada.* May 20, p. 4.

"Exonera Publicamente EU al Sistema Bancária Mexicano." 1998. *Excelsiór, El Periódico de la Vida Nacionál.* May 22, p. 10-A.

Fineberg, Harvey V. 1988. Education to Prevent AIDS: Prospects and Obstacles. *Science,* 239(2):592-596.

Fitzsimmons, Pamela. 1999. "SB Judge Makes Injunction Against Prostitutes Permanent." *San Bernardino County Sun,* March 12, p. B3.

Flanigan, James. 1998. "San Bernardino Shows Comeback Spunk." *Los Angeles Times,* August 1, p. D1.

Fleming, Patricia L., P. A. Sweeney, R.L. Frey, M.A. Mays, and J.W. Ward. 1998. "AIDS Surveillance Trends in the United States: Declines in AIDS Diagnoses and Deaths Direct a Shift to Integrated HIV/AIDS Case Surveillance." *12th World AIDS Conference, Abstracts-on-Disk.* Whitehouse Station, NJ: Merck and Co.

Flynn, Neil M., S. Jane, S. Harper, V. Bailey, R. Anderson, and G. Acuna. 1987. "Sharing of Paraphernalia in Intravenous Drug Users (IVDU): Knowledge of AIDS is Incomplete and Doesn't Affect Behavior." *III International Conference on AIDS. Abstracts Volume.* Washington, DC: U.S. Department of Health and Human Services.

Friedman, Samuel R. and Douglas S. Lipton. 1991. Editorial. In Samuel R. Friedman, Douglas S. Lipton, and Barry Stimmel (Eds.), *Cocaine, AIDS, and Intravenous Drug Use* (pp. 18-22). Binghamton, NY: The Haworth Press.

Gaza, Adolfo. 1999. "Mexican Police Seek Respect." *San Bernardino County Sun,* April 8, p. A14.

Geeta, Bhave, Christina P. Lindan, and Esther S. Hudes. 1995. Impact of an Intervention on HIV, Sexually Transmitted Diseases, and Condom Use Among Sex Workers in Bombay, India. *AIDS,* 9(suppl.1): 521-530.

Ghys, Peter, Guessan Mah-Bi, M. Traore, Y. Konan, B. Vuylsteke, A. Tiemele, K. Kale, O. Tawil, I.M. Coulibaly, S.Z. Wiktor, et al. 1998. "Trends in Condom Use Between 1991 and 1997 and Obstacles to 100 Percent Condom Use in Female Sex Workers (FSW) in Abidjan, Cote d'Ivoire." *12th World AIDS Conference, Abstracts-on-Disk.* Whitehouse Station, NJ: Merck and Co.

Goldstein, Avram. 1970. Urine Testing Schedules in Methadone Maintenance Treatment of Heroin Addiction. *Journal of the American Medical Association,* 210(October 12): 311.

Govindaraj, Sanjay, Sanjav Govindaraj, and Dhananjay Appachu. 1998. "Medical Care and HIV/AIDS Prevention for Children in Sex Work—Bangalore, India." *12th World AIDS Conference, Abstracts-on-Disk.* Whitehouse Station, NJ: Merck and Co.

Hagan, Elizabeth and Joan Gormley, 1998. *HIV and the Drug Culture.* Binghamton, NY: The Haworth Press.

Hagan, Holly, Peter Gupton, Gary Tompkins, Walter Harris, and James Smith. 1991. The Tacoma Syringe Exchange. In Samuel R. Friedman, Douglas S. Lipton, and Barry Stimmel (Eds.) *Cocaine, AIDS, and Intravenous Drug Abuse* (pp. 81-88). Binghamton, NY: The Haworth Press.

Hartigan, Pamela. 1994. The Response of Nongovernmental Organizations in Latin America to HV Infection and AIDS: A Vehicle for Grasping the Contributions NGOs Make to Health and Development. In Douglas A. Feldman (Ed.), *Global AIDS Policy* (pp. 47-60). Westport, CT: Bergin and Garvey.

Haynes, Karima. 2000. "'Babydol' Gets 3-Year Prison Term." *Los Angeles Times,* May 16, p. B3.

Henriques, Fernando. 1963. *Prostitution in Society: A Survey.* New York: Citadel Press.

"HepC, Thriving on Ignorance." 2000. *Los Angeles Times.* Editorial. July 16, p. B4.

Herbert, Bob. 2001. "A Missing AIDS Lifeline." *Liberal Opinion Week,* July 16, 2001.

Hodding, Glenn, Michael Jann, and Irving Ackerman. 1980. Drug Withdrawal Syndromes: A Literature Review. *Western Journal of Medicine.* 133 (November): 383-391.

Hosobuchi, Yoshio, John E. Adams, and Rita Linchitz. 1977. Pain Relief by Electrical Stimulation of the Central Gray Matter in Humans and Its Reversal by Naloxone. *Science* 197(July 8): 183-186.

Ignoto, Barbara. 1999. *Confessions of a Part-Time Call Girl.* New York: Verso.

"Injunction Best Tack for SB Prostitute Problem." 2001. *San Bernardino County Sun,* Editorial. June 2, p. B7.

James, Jennifer. 1976. Motivations for Entrance into Prostitution. In Laura Grites (Ed.), *The Female Offender* (pp. 177-205). Lexington, Mass.: Lexington Books.

Kaplan, John. 1983. *The Hardest Drug: Heroin and Public Policy.* Chicago: The University of Chicago Press.

Koop, C. Everett. 1986. *Surgeon General's Report on Acquired Immune Deficiency Syndrome.* Washington, DC: U.S. Department of Health and Human Services.

Krasnowski, Matt. 1999. "3 convictions End Operation Casablanca." *The San Diego Union-Tribune,* December 21, p. A-4.

Kreiss, Joan K., Davy Koech, Francis A. Plummer, King K. Holmes, Marilyn Lightfoote, Peter Piot, Allan R. Ronald, Ndinya-Achola, Lourdes J. D'Costa, Racia Roberts, et al. 1986. AIDS Virus Infection in Nairobi Prostitutes: Spread of the Epidemic to East Africa. *New England Journal of Medicine,* 314(2): 414-418.

Lait, Matt and Shawn Hubler. 1999. "Investigation of Prostitution Ring Attracts IRS Interest." *Los Angeles Times,* June 12, p. B1.

"Lavaron Once Bancos 55 Milliones de Dólares." 1998. *Reforma.* May 20, p. 4-A.

Levine, Michael. 1998. *The Big White Lie: The Deep Cover Operation That Exposed the CIA Sabotage of the Drug War.* New York: Thunder's Mouth.

Lewis, Diana. 1985. *The Prostitute and Her Clients: Your Pleasure is Her Business.* Springfield, IL.: Charles C. Thomas.

*The Living New Testament.* 1967. Wheaton, IL: Tyndale House.

Lopez, Sonny. 1998. "Ex-Juarez Mayor Favored in Chihuahua Elections." *El Paso Times,* March 30, 1998.

Los Angeles County Department of Health Services. 1987. Recommendations for Prevention of AIDS Transmission in Health Care Settings. *Public Health Letter,* 9(11), November.

———. 1997. Reported Communicable Diseases. *Public Health Letter,* 19(2), March.

_____. 1998a. Reported Communicable Diseases. *Public Health Letter.* 20(6), July/August.

_____. 1998b. Reported Communicable Diseases. *Public Health Letter.* 20(8), October.

_____. 1999a. Reported Communicable Diseases. *Public Health Letter.* 21(3), April.

_____. 1999b. Reported Communicable Diseases. *Public Health Letter,* 21(10), December.

_____. 2000. Reported Communicable Diseases. *Public Health Letter.* 22(1), January.

Lurie, Peter G., E. Drucker, and A. Knowles. 1998. Still Working After All These Years: Increasing Evidence of Needle Exchange Program (NEP) Effectiveness in Studies Published Since 1993. *12th World AIDS Conference, Abstracts-on-Disk.* Whitehouse Station, NJ: Merck and Co.

Macella, Gabriel and Donald Schulz. 1997. "Mexico: Will a Larger Military Role Harm Democracy?" *Los Angeles Times.* January 19, p. M2.

Madge, John. 1965. *The Tools of Social Science.* New York: Doubleday Anchor.

Mahmud, Hasan, M.A. Kabir, M.A.H. Mian, and E. Karim. 1998. Behavioral Risk Assessment and Serology for Syphilis, Hepatitis B and HIV Among Commercial Sex Workers in an Isolated Brothel in Coalanda, Rajbari. *12th World AIDS Conference, Abstracts-on-Disk.* Whitehouse Station, NJ: Merck and Co.

Maingot, Anthony P. 1988. Laundering the Gains of the Drug Trade: Miami and Caribbean Tax Havens. *Journal of Interamerican Studies and World Affairs,* 30:2-3: 181.

Martinez, Angelica. 2001. "Prostitution: Never-ending headache." *San Bernardino County Sun,* July 30, p. A1.

Martinez, Carlos Lopez, C. Magiz-Rodríguez, and P. Uribe-Zunga. 1998. "Kaposi's Sarcoma in AIDS Mexican patients." *12th World AIDS Conference, Abstracts-on-Disk.* Whitehouse Station, NJ: Merck and Co.

Martinez, Oscar J. 1994. *Border People: Life and Society in the U.S.-Mexican Borderlands.* University of Arizona Press.

Maugh, Thomas H. II. 1998. "Heroin Use Soars in State, Study Says." *Los Angeles Times,* July 11, p. A1.

Mavromataki, Maria. 1997. *Greek Mythology and Religion.* Athens: Haitalis Press.

McAuliffe, William E., S. Doering, P. Breer, H. Silverman, B. Branson, and K. Williams. 1987. An Evaluation of Using Ex-Addict Outreach Workers to Educate Intravenous Drug Users About AIDS Prevention. *III International Conference on AIDS. Abstracts Volume.* Washington, DC: U.S. Department of Health and Human Services.

McCoy, Alfred W. 1972. *The Politics of Heroin in Southeast Asia.* New York: Harper and Row.

McDonnell, Patrick, Ken Ellingwood, and Hector Tobar. 1998. "Officials Link Ensenada Massacre to Drug Feud." *Los Angeles Times,* September 19, p. A1.

McLellan, A. Thomas, Charles Winick, William Schumer, and Martha Thompson. 1993. The Effects of Psychosocial Services in Substance Abuse Treatment. *Journal of the American Medical Association,* 269(April 21): 1953-1959.

"México no es Narcoestado." 1998. *Excelsiór, El Periódico de la Vida Nacionál.* May 6, p. 26-A.

"Mexico Sting Irks Secretary," 1998. *Albuquerque Journal.* June 13, p. A-3.

Millett, Kate. 1971. *The Prostitution Papers: "A Quartet for Female Voice."* New York: Ballantine Books.

Millman, Joel. 1996. "Asian Investment Floods Into Mexican Border Region." *The Wall Street Journal,* September 6, p. A10.

Mondragon, Raul Ortiz, A. Ruiz-Badillo, C. Magis-Rodriguez, R. Lozada, R. Ramos, J.B. Ferreira-Pinto, and M.E. Ramos. 1998. "HIV Risk Transmission in Mexican Injecting Women." *12th World AIDS Conference, Abstracts-on-Disk.* Whitehouse Station, NJ: Merck and Co.

Musto, David. 1973. *The American Disease: Origins of Narcotic Control.* New Haven: Yale University Press.

Nadelmann, Ethan A. 1988. The Case for Legalization. 1988. *The Public Interest,* 92(Summer): 3-31.

*The Nation.* 1998. Classified, January 9, p. 34.

National Commission on AIDS. 1993. *Financing Health Care for Persons with HIV Disease: Policy Options - Technical Report Prepared for the National Commission on AIDS.* Washington, DC: U.S. Department of Health and Human Services.

Nazario, Sonia. 1999. "Sobering Facts." *Los Angeles Times,* March 21, p. A1.

Neergaard, Lauran. 1998. "Treating Addicts Works, Cuts, Doctors Say." *The Arizona Republic,* March 18, p. A-4.

New York City Health Department. 1920. *The New York City Narcotic Clinic.* New York: Bureau of Public Health Education, Health Department.

"Niegan Registro a Sindicato de Prostitutas." 1998. *Excelsiór, El Periódico de la Vida Nacionál.* May 11, p. 19-A.

"No Coinciden con la Información de Semafa. Muertos Subitas." 1998. *Excelsiór, El Periódico de la Vida Nacionál.* May 11, p.28.

Noll, Danielle R. 1996. Solving the Problem of Threats to Care for Medicaid Beneficiaries with HIV/AIDS. *Policy Perspectives: George Washington University Journal of Public Administration,* 3 (1): 9-21.

"No To Re-Opening Narcotics Clinic." 1938. *San Francisco Examiner.* December 17, p. C-1.

Novick, Leonard F., Donald Berns, Rachel Stricof, Roy Stevens, Kenneth Pass, and Judith Wethers. 1989. HIV Seroprevalence in Newborns in New York State. *Journal of the American Medical Association,* 261 (1):1745-1750.

Nzilambi, Nzila, Kevin M. DeCock, Donald N. Forthal, Henry Francis, Robert W. Ryder, Ismey Malebe, Jane Getchell, Marie Laga, Peter Piot, and Joseph B. McCormick. 1988. The Prevalence of Infection With Human Immunodeficiency

Virus Over a Ten-Year Period in Rural Zaire. *New England Journal of Medicine*, 318(February 4):276-279.

O'Connor, Anne-Marie. 1996a. "Epidemic of Drug-Related Murders Plagues Tijuana." *Los Angeles Times*, September 10, p. A1.

_____. 1996b. "Tijuana Scions of Privilege Alleged to Be Drug Hit Men." *Los Angeles Times,*. November 13, p. A-1.

_____. 1998. "Mexico's City of Promise." *Los Angeles Times*, January 1, p. A-1.

Ojeda de la Peña, Norma and Gudélia Rangel. 1996. "Maternal Health Among Working Women: A Case Study in the Mexican-U.S. Border." *Estudios Fronterizos*, 37-38(Enero-junio/julio-diciembre): 33-60.

Olch, Peter D. 1975. William S. Halsted and Local Anesthesia: Contributions and Complications. *Anesthesiology*, 42 (April): 479-486.

Papaevengelou, G., A. Roumeliotou-Karayannis, G. Kallinikos, and G. Papoutsakis. 1985. LAV/HTLV-III Infection in Female Prostitutes. Letter. *The Lancet* II(November 2): 1018.

Paternostro, Silvana. 1995. Mexico as a Narco-Democracy. *World Policy Journal*, (Spring): 1-7.

Phederson, G. (Ed.). 1989. *A Vindication of the Rights of Whores*. Seattle: Seal Press.

Pick, James B. and Edgar W. Butler. 1997. *Mexico Megacity*. Boulder: Westview Press.

Piot, Peter, Francis A. Plummer, Fred S. Mhalu, Jean-Louis Lamboray, James Chin, and Jonathan M. Mann. 1988. AIDS: An International Perspective. *Science*, 239 (February 5): 573-579.

Platt, Leah. 2001. Stopping at a Red Light. *The Nation*, July 9, pp. 40-42.

"Posición del PAN hácia el 2000." 1998. *Diário de Morelos*. May 12, p. 2.

Quinn, Thomas C., Jonathan M. Mann, James W. Curran, and Peter Piot. 1986. AIDS in Africa: An Epidemiologic Paradigm. *Science*, 234(November 21): 955-963.

Ravitch, Mark M. 1986. Dr. Halsted's Hernia. *Surgery*. 100(July): 59-67.

Read, Jodi Ohlsen. 1999. It isn't Over Yet: AIDS. *Medical Bulletin*, University of Minnesota, Spring: 12-15.

Regier, Darrel A. and M.E. Farmer. (1990). Comorbidity of Mental Disorders With Alcohol and Other Drug Abuse: Results from the Epidemiologic Catchment Area (ECA) Study. *Journal of the American Medical Association*, 264(November 21): 2511-2518.

Reinarman, Craig and Harry G. Levine. 1998. *Crack in America: Demon Drugs and Social Justice*. Berkeley: University of California Press.

Roane, Kit R. 1998. "Prostitutes on Wane In New York Streets But Take to Internet." *The New York Times*, February 23, pp. 3-1.

Rodríguez, Carlos Magis, E. Bravo Garcia, E. Rodriguez Nolasco, and P.E. Uribe Zuniga. 1998a. Rural AIDS cases in Mexico. *12th World AIDS Conference, Abstracts-on-Disk*. Whitehouse Station, NJ: Merck and Co.

Rodríguez, Carlos Magis, A. Ruiz-Badillo, R.E. Loo Mendez, M. Santarriaga Sandoval, and P.E. Uribe Zuniga. 1998b. "Sentinel Studies In Intravenous Drug Users in Mexico." *12th World AIDS Conference, Abstracts-on-Disk.* Whitehouse Station, NJ: Merck and Co.

Root-Bernstein, Robert S. 1996. Misleading Reliability, *Scientific American,* 274(2): 6-8.

Rosas, Solís A., G. Rangel, and J. Diaz. 1996. "Social Factors of Female Prostituting That Influence on Their Health Condition: HIV and Sexually Transmitted Diseases. The Case of Tijuana, B.C., Mexico." *XI International Conference on AIDS, Abstracts-on-Disk.* Whitehouse Station, NJ: Merck and Co.

Rosenzweig, David. 1999a. "4 to Testify in Cross-Border Money Laundering Case." *Los Angeles Times,* January 9, 1999, p. B1.

_____. 1999b. "Key Figure in Cartel Case Pleads Guilty." *Los Angeles Times,* March 9, p. B1.

Rotello, Gabriel. 1996. "The Twilight of AIDS?" *The Nation,* December 23, pp. 16-20.

Russell, Dick. 1998. Poetry in Motion: Homero Aridjis, Mexico's Environmental Conscience, Fuses Literature and Activism. Natural Resources Defense Council. *The Amicus Journal* (Fall): 34-37.

Sabatier, Renee C. 1987. Social, Cultural and Demographic Aspects of AIDS. *Western Journal of Medicine* [Special Issue—AIDS—A Global Perspective], 147(December):713-715.

"Salinas Kin Linked to Cocaine." 1998. *Los Angeles Times.* September 20, p. A8.

San Bernardino County, 2001. *AIDS Program Report: AIDS/HIV Disease Reported Through December 31, 1999.* San Bernardino, California: San Bernardino County Department of Public Health.

San Bernardino Countywide Gangs and Drugs Task Force, 1998. Minutes of statement by San Bernardino County District Attorney Dennis Stout at Gangs and Drugs Task Force meeting, July 8.

Sanchez, Roberto. 1990. Condiciones de vida de los trabajadores de la maquiladora en Tijuana y Nogales. *Frontera norte,* 2(July-December).

"San Diego Will Tell GOP Cross-Border Success Story." 1996. *Statesman Journal,* July 24, p. A-2.

Sandovál, Martha Santarriaga, R.E. Loo Mendez, C. Magis Rodriguez, and P.E. Uribe Zuniga. 1998. "Female Sex Workers in Mexico: Sentinel Surveillance 1990-1997." *12th World AIDS Conference, Abstracts-on-Disk.* Whitehouse Station, NJ: Merck and Co.

Sankary, Timothy, R. Frerichs, M. Kihara, M. Miyao, K. Nakajima, and K. Tadokoro. 1998. "HIV Risk Behavior Intervention Trial in Foreign Female Prostitutes (FFPs) in Japan." *12th World AIDS Conference, Abstracts-on-Disk.* Whitehouse Station, NJ: Merck and Co.

Selwyn, Peter A. 1988. Sterile Needles and the Epidemic of Acquired Immunodeficiency Syndrome: Issues for Drug Abuse Treatment and Public Health. In Larry

Siegel (Ed.), *AIDS and Substance Abuse* (pp. 99-106). Binghamton, NY: The Haworth Press.

Shapiro, Walter. 1975. The Two Party Pork Barrel. *The Washington Monthly,* (April): pp. 24-30.

Sheridan, Mary Beth. 1996. "Baja Drug Prosecutor Replaced Amid Killings." *Los Angeles Times,* October 2, p. A-3.

_____. 1998a. "Alleged Pioneer of Mexico-U.S. Cocaine Trade Found Slain." *Los Angeles Times,* September 12, p. A3.

_____. 1998b. "Drug Turf War Takes Toll on City." *Los Angeles Times,* February 28, p. A1.

_____. 1998c. "Traffickers Move Into Yucatan Peninsula." *Los Angeles Times,* August 27, p. A1.

_____. 1999. "Mexican Ex-Governor Flees to Avoid Jail." *Los Angeles Times,* April 7, p. A23.

_____. 2000. "Juarez Mayor Wages Own War on Drug Cartel." *Los Angeles Times,* February 2, p. A1.

Sheridan, Mary Beth and Annie-Marie O'Connor. 1996. "Slaying of Tijuana Prosecutor Spurs Renewed Uproar Over Conspiracies." *Los Angeles Times,* August 21, p. A1.

Sheridan, Mary Beth and James F. Smith. 1999. "Raul Salinas Gets 50 Years for Murder." *Los Angeles Times,* January 22, p. A1.

Smith, Carla Dillard, Gloria Lockett, and Michael Bala. 1996. "Prostitutes: Their HIV Knowledge and Condom Use." *XI International Conference on AIDS, Abstracts-on-Disk.* Whitehouse Station, NJ: Merck and Co.

Smith, Gregory L. 1986. Lack of HIV Infection and Condom Use in Licensed Prostitutes. *Lancet,* 139(4): 1392

Smith, James F. 2001. "Father Hailed for Taking Justice Into His Own Hands." *Los Angeles Times,* June 6, p. A1.

Solís, Dianne. 1996. "Rich Tijuana Youths Major in Narcotics." *The Wall Street Journal,* November 7, p. A16.

Sonnenreich, Michael R. 1973. Discussion of the Final Report of the National Commission on Marijuana and Drug Abuse. *Villanova Law Review,* 18(May): 818.

Sorensen, James L. and Amy L. Copeland. 2000. Drug Abuse Treatment as an HIV Prevention Strategy: A Review. *Drug and Alcohol Dependence* 59(2000): 17-31.

"State Should Not Take Over Selling Dope." 1938. *Seattle Post-Intelligencer.* February 17, p. 22.

Stein, Carl. 1993. Peripheral Mechanisms of Opioid Analgesia. *Anesthesia and Analgesia,* 76(1): 182-91.

Stevens, Charles, S. Norman, M. Shaukat, K. Nay, J. Herbst, and M. Cohn. 1986. Human T-Cell Lymphotropic Virus Type III Infection in a Cohort of Homosexual Men in New York City. *Journal of the American Medical Association* 255 (December 2): 2167-2172.

Stockman, David A. 1975. The Social Pork Barrel. *The Public Interest,* 15(Spring): 3-30.

Symanski, Richard. 1981. *The Immoral Landscape: Female Prostitution in Western Societies.* Toronto: Butterworth and Company.

Texeira, Erin. 2000. "Justice is Not Color Blind." *Los Angeles Times,* May 22, p. B1.

Thomas, Pete. 1998. "Baja Attacks Raise Concerns About the Safety of Travelers." *Los Angeles Times,* January 16, p. C-8.

Tirelli, Umberto, Emanuela Vaccher, Antonio Carbone, Paolo De Paoli, GianFranco Santini, and Silvio Monfardini. 1985. "HTLV-III Antibody in Prostitutes." Letter. *The Lancet* II(December 21/28): 1424.

Toro, Maria Celia. 1995. *Mexico's "War" on Drugs: Causes and Consequences.* Boulder, CO: Lynne Rienner Publishers.

Trebach, Arnold S. 1982. *The Heroin Solution.* New Haven: Yale University Press.

"Turistas Extranjeros Sufran en la Capitál mas de 3 Robos Diários Con Violéncia." 1998. *Excelsiór, El Periódico de la Vida Nacionál.* May 11, p. 1-A.

U.S. Commissioner of Internal Revenue. 1921. *Annual Report of the Commissioner of Internal Revenue for the Fiscal Year 1920.* Washington, DC: U.S. Government Printing Office.

U.S. Department of Health and Human Services. 1997. "Needle Exchange Programs in America: Review of Published Studies and Ongoing Research." Report to the Committee on Appropriations for the Department of Labor, Health and Human Services, Education and Related Agencies. Washington, DC: U.S. Government Printing Office.

U.S. Department of Justice, Office of Justice Programs, Bureau of Justice Statistics. 1997. *Crime in the United States 1996.* Washington, DC: U.S. Government Printing Office.

———. 1998. *Bulletin.* "Census of State and Local Law Enforcement Agencies, 1996." Author.

———. 1999. "Local Police Departments, 1997." Author.

Valenstein, Elliot S. 1978. "Science-Fiction Fantasy and the Brain." *Psychology Today,* July, pp. 29-39.

Van De Perre, Marjorie Rober-Guroff, Pierre Freyens, Robert C. Gallo, Nathan Clumeck, Elie Nzabihimana, Partrick De Mol, Jean-Paul Butzler, Jean-Baptiste Kanyamupira. 1985. Female Prostitutes: A Risk Group For Infection With Human T-Cell Lymphotropic Virus Type III. *The Lancet* II(September 7): 524-527.

Vargas, Galileo. 1998. "Medical Students Mobilize to Provide Information to a Whole University Community." *12th World AIDS Conference, Abstracts-on-Disk.* Whitehouse Station, NJ: Merck and Co.

Velasco-Hernandez, Jorge X. 1997. "Modeling HIV Prevalence Among Female Prostitutes in Tijuana." Paper presented at 1997 International Conference on Mathematical Models in Medical and Health Sciences, Madrid, April, 14.

Velóz, Patricia, M.L. Coeto, and L. Villegas. 1998. "HIV/AIDS Knowledge Among Rural Women in Mexico." *12th World AIDS Conference, Abstracts-on-Disk.* Whitehouse Station, NJ: Merck and Co.

Vlahov, David, C. Flynn, R. Brookmeyer, B. Junge, M. Safaeian, P. Beilenson, and K.E. Nelson. 1998. "Lower Risk of HIV Infection with Continued Regular Participation in Needle Exchange Programs." *12th World AIDS Conference, Abstracts-on-Disk.* Whitehouse Station, NJ: Merck and Co.

Vogt, Marcus W., Donald E. Craven, David F. Crawford, David J. Witt, Roy Byington, Robert Schooley, and Martin S. Hirsch. 1986. Isolation of HTLV-III/LAV From Cervical Secretions of Women at Risk for AIDS. *The Lancet,* II(March): 525-527.

Von Bargen, Jennifer, K.S. Miller, S. Faruque, C. Word, C.B. McCoy, and B.R. Edlin. 1998. "HIV Infection and Risk Behavior Among Urban Female Sex Workers: Missed Opportunities for Intervention." *12th World AIDS Conference, Abstracts-on-Disk.* Whitehouse Station, NJ: Merck and Co.

Von Reyn, C. Fordham and Jonathan M. Mann. 1987. Global Epidemiology. *Western Journal of Medicine* [Special Issue, AIDS—A Global Perspective], 147 (6): 694-701.

Walker, William O. 1981. *Drug Control in the Americas.* Albuquerque: University of New Mexico Press.

Wallace, J.I., D. Bloch, R. Whitmore, M. Cushing, and A. Weiner. 1996. "Fellatio is a Significant Risk Activity for Acquiring AIDS in New York City (NYC) Streetwalking Sex Workers." *XI Internacional Conference on AIDS, Abstracts-on-Disk.* Whitehouse Station, NJ: Merck and Co.

Wallace, J.I., P.J. Alexander, S.R. Horn, A. Weiner, M. Hidalgo, and L. Dolphus. 1998. "Give Them What They Need, and They'll Keep Coming Back for More, Reducing the Incidence of HIV Among Female, Streetbased Sex Workers in New York City." *12th World AIDS Conference, Abstracts-on-Disk.* Whitehouse Station, NJ: Merck and Co.

Wallich, Paul. 1989. AIDS Counts: Planning for an Epidemic Whose Size Still Counts. *Scientific American,* 267(4): 17-18.

Wangensteen, Owen N. and Sarah Wangensteen. 1978. *The Rise of Surgery: Empiric Craft to Scientific Discipline.* Minneapolis: University of Minnesota Press.

Watters, John K. 1987. "Preventing Human Immunodeficiency Virus Contagion Among Intravenous Drug Users: The Impact of Street-Based Education on Risk-Behavior." *III International Conference on AIDS. Abstracts Volume.* Washington, DC: U.S. Department of Health and Human Services.

Webb, Gary. 1998. *Dark Alliance: The CIA, the Contras, and the Crack Cocaine Explosion.* New York: Seven Stories.

Wiebel, W. Wayne, Antonio Jinenez, Wendell Johnson, Lawrence Ouellet, Borko Jovanovic, Thomas Lampinen, James Murray, and Mary Utne O'Brien. 1996. Risk Behavior and HIV Seroincidence Among Out-of-Treatment Injection Drug Users: A Four-Year Prospective Study. *Journal of Acquired Immune Deficiency Syndromes and Human Retrovirology,* 12(3): 282-289.

Williams, Ann, H. Wolf, C. You, and M. Singh. 1998. "Adherence to Antiretroviral Therapy Among HIV Positive Women." *12th World AIDS Conference, Abstracts-on-Disk.* Whitehouse Station, NJ: Merck and Co.

Williams, Carol. 1999. "Germany's Prostitutes May Get Social Benefits." *Los Angeles Times,* October 21, p. A12.

Winick, Charles C. and Paul M. Kinsie. 1971. *Prostitution in the United States.* New York: Quadrangle Books.

Winik, Lyric Wallwork. 2000. "He Has A Better Way." *Parade Magazine,* January 16, pp. 4-6.

Wisnia, Steven. 2001. "New Drug Bizarre: Bush Picks Ex-Bennett Aide as Drug Czar." *High Times,* August, p. 24.

Wofsy, Carl B. 1988. Women and the Acquired Immunodeficiency Syndrome: An Interview. *Western Journal of Medicine,* 149: 687-690.

Woody, George E., A.T. McLellan, and C.P. O'Brien. 1983. Psychotherapy for Opiate Addicts: Does It Help? *Archives of General Psychiatry,* 40(June): 639-645.

Woody, George E., C.P. O'Brien, F. Zackson, and W.E. McAuliffe. 1986. Psychotherapy for Substance Abuse. *Psychiatric Clinics of North America,* 9(September): 547-562.

Zausner, Michael. 1986. *The Streets: A Factual Portrait of Six Prostitutes as Told in Their Own Words.* New York: St. Martin's Press.

Zweben, Joan Ellen, 1991. Counseling Issues in Methadone Maintenance Treatment. *Journal of Psychoactive Drugs,* 23(April-June): 177-190.

# Index

Page numbers followed by the letter "f" indicate figures; those followed by the letter "t" indicate tables.